Souha Hannachi
Khaoula Saadani
Rym Abid

Osteoarticular brucellosis

Souha Hannachi
Khaoula Saadani
Rym Abid

Osteoarticular brucellosis

ScienciaScripts

Imprint

Cover image: www.ingimage.com

This book is a translation from the original published under ISBN 978-620-6-70793-6.

Publisher:
Sciencia Scripts
is a trademark of
Dodo Books Indian Ocean Ltd. and OmniScriptum S.R.L publishing group

120 High Road, East Finchley, London, N2 9ED, United Kingdom
Str. Armeneasca 28/1, office 1, Chisinau MD-2012, Republic of Moldova, Europe
Printed at: see last page
ISBN: 978-620-7-68286-7

Introduction

Brucellosis, historically known as "Malta fever", "melitococcie" or "Mediterranean undulant fever", is one of the world's most widespread anthropozoonoses (1). Worldwide incidence is estimated at 500,000 human cases per year (2).

Brucella are small, intracellular, aerobic, gram-negative, non-motile, non-spore-forming coccobacilli that can only reproduce intracellularly(3).

The reservoir is animal, mainly affecting livestock species. There are eight main species: *B. abortus, B. melitensis, B. suis, B. ovis, B. canis, B. neotomae, B. cetaceae and B. pinnipediae.*

The most important species for humans are *B. melitensis, B. abortus and B. suis*, which share over 90% sequence identity.

B. melitensis is the most virulent species, responsible for the most serious infections.

Epidemiologically, brucellosis has become rare in developed countries, thanks to a stringent policy of screening and eradication of the animal disease, notably through vaccination and slaughter of infected animals. However, it remains endemic in most underdeveloped countries, notably those of the Mediterranean basin, the Middle East, West Asia, Africa and Latin America, where it causes major economic losses and poses a serious threat to human health(2,3,6-8).

In Tunisia, brucellosis is a notifiable disease. Epidemiological surveillance is organized by the Directorate of Basic Health Care (DSSB) under the supervision of the Ministry of Health and the Ministry of Agriculture (5). The disease is endemic mainly in central-western and southern Tunisia. Prior to 1989, endemicity was low. In fact, the annual average number of cases reported was 5. Slacker preventive measures and the introduction of infected animals from neighboring countries were at the root of the 1991-1992 epidemic, which totaled over 500 cases in the south-western regions(6). Since the introduction of government vaccination of small ruminants (sheep and cattle), the incidence of the disease has stabilized until 2013. Since then, there has been a gradual increase in incidence, from 0.14 cases/100,000 inhabitants to 0.99 cases/100,000 inhabitants in 2018, corresponding to a more than 7-fold increase. The highest annual incidence of human brucellosis was recorded in 2017, with 1.13 cases/100,000 inhabitants (10).

Brucellosis can be transmitted directly or indirectly to humans. In the majority of cases, transmission is indirect, via the food chain, following ingestion of raw milk or its derivatives (especially fromage frais) from infected animals. Cow's, ewe's, goat's, buffalo's and camel's milk are the main *Brucella-carrying* foodstuffs consumed raw. This mode of transmission is considered the main route of contamination in both urban and rural areas.

Humans can also become directly infected through contact with infected animals, mainly via the mucocutaneous route, and rarely via the respiratory route following inhalation of infected dust. Sexual or transplacental contamination is exceptional.

Mucocutaneous contamination is more frequent in rural areas and among professionally exposed people. It affects people handling the products of abortions or the births of infected animals(7).

In fact, brucellosis is considered an occupational hazard for people working in the livestock sector. They come into contact with blood, placenta, foetuses and uterine secretions, and run a greater risk of contracting the disease. This method of transmission mainly affects farmers, butchers, hunters, veterinarians and laboratory staff.

As humans are secondary or accidental hosts, there is no human-to-human transmission.

Clinically speaking, human brucellosis is a multi-systemic disease causing septicemia via the lymphatic system, with extremely polymorphous and non-specific clinical manifestations. After a silent incubation period averaging 15 days, the first symptoms of the acute phase generally appear progressively. Symptoms include persistent asthenia, headache, undulating fever typically associated with profuse night sweats, and muscle and joint pain. Clinical examination is often normal, although hepatomegaly, splenomegaly and small adenopathies may be present(8,9).

The disease then evolves towards a focal phase marked by the appearance of secondary localizations, essentially osteoarticular, neuromeningeal or cardiac. Other hepatosplenic or genital localizations remain possible. The chronic form, defined by a prolonged course lasting more than a year, is responsible for physical, intellectual and sexual asthenia(3,10-12).

Human brucellosis is a multi-systemic disease with a broad spectrum of clinical manifestations, which can lead to delayed diagnosis and treatment, with an increased risk of developing complications(13,14).

The aim of our work was to study the epidemiological, clinical, microbiological and therapeutic features of osteoarticular brucellosis.

Methods

1. Type of study:

This was a descriptive, retrospective, observational, single-center study conducted in the Infectious Diseases Department of the Hôpital Militaire Principal d'Instruction de Tunis, covering patients with brucellosis in all clinical forms over a 15-year period from January 2008 to December 2022.

2. Population:

In order to have a homogeneous population and minimize possible biases, we established inclusion, non-inclusion and exclusion criteria.

2.1 Inclusion criteria:

We included all patients aged 18 years hospitalized for osteoarticular brucellosis:

- An epidemiological context suggestive of brucellian origin:

Consumption of unpasteurized dairy products, participation in farrowing or milking, mastitis or abortion in the herd, or a high-risk occupation.

- A clinical history suggestive of acute septicemic brucellosis (ASB), either focal or chronic.

- In focalized forms, imaging to confirm focalization.

- And microbiological confirmation by:

- Isolation of *Brucella* spp in blood cultures or other biological samples (joint fluid, abscess pus, etc.) and/or

- Positive brucellosis serology: Rose Bengal test (RB) or Wright seroagglutination (SW)

2.2 Non-inclusion criteria:

Patients with no microbiological confirmation of brucellosis.

Patients with another clinical form of brucellosis (acute, organ-focused or chronic).

2.3 Exclusion criteria:

We excluded all patients whose available data were deemed insufficient or who were lost to follow-up before completing explorations and/or therapeutic management.

3. Course of the study:

The main source of data was the contents of medical records, the transfer letters.

The data collected was reported on a data sheet based on recent studies in the literature (Appendix 1).

4. Definition of variables and measuring instruments:

4.1 Epidemiological study:

The various parameters assessed were:

- Patient's age at diagnosis;
- gender, geographic origin;
- the profession;
- Comorbidities and history;
- Risk factors and predisposing circumstances: consumption of unpasteurized raw milk and its by-products, participation in calving and/or milking the herd;
- Reason for admission, consultation and diagnosis times, and length of hospital stay;
- Functional and physical signs: fever, sweats, arthralgia, myalgia, chills, sciatica, spinal pain, hip pain, buttock pain, neurological disorder, asthenia, anorexia, weight loss, hepatomegaly, splenomegaly, adenopathy, orchitis, behavioral disorder, meningeal syndrome;
- The clinical form chosen, and the site for the focal form.

4.2 Further tests:

4.2.1 Routine biological tests:

-Complete blood count (CBC),

-Transaminases,

-Cholestasis markers,

-Urea/creatinine,

-Ionogram,

-Total protein/albumin,

-C-reactive protein (CRP), sedimentation rate (VS).

4.2.2 Microbiological tests:

-Blood cultures,

-Brucellosis serology (Rose Bengal (RB) test and Wright serodiagnosis (SW)).

-Indirect immunofluorescence (IFI)

-Polymerase Chain Reaction (PCR) on biological fluid (joint fluid, pus, etc.).

4.2.3 Radiological examinations:

Standard X-rays,

-Computed tomography (CT)

-Magnetic resonance imaging (MRI)

-Soft tissue ultrasound

4.3 Therapeutic parameters:

4.3.1 Antibiotic treatment:

We specified the molecules prescribed, the dosage and the method of administration, essentially according to clinical form. In addition, adjuvant treatment was necessary in several cases.

4.3.2 Adjuvant treatment:

Adjuvant treatment including corticosteroid therapy, curative or preventive anticoagulation or immobilization was noted in this study.

4.3.3 Duration of treatment:

We noted the duration of treatment. This varied according to the patient's clinical form, site and terrain.

Compliance and clinico-biological tolerance of treatment were noted.

4.3.4 Surgical treatment:

We have specified the types and indications of surgical treatment for certain patients.

4.4 Clinical course:

4.4.1 Length of hospital stay:

The duration of hospitalization was counted in days from the patient's admission to discharge.

4.4.2 Disease complications and progression:

We looked for any decompensation of a tare or appearance of a complication secondary to the infection, such as the appearance of a neurological disorder or decompensation of a tare.

Cure of brucellosis is usually determined by the absence of clinical symptoms, normalization of inflammatory markers in blood tests, and absence of progression of radiological lesions.

The persistence of pain or any type of deficit at the end of treatment constitutes a sequel.

A relapse of brucellosis is generally defined by the reappearance of clinical symptoms suggestive of the disease or the re-isolation of *Brucella* from the second month or after the end of initial treatment.

Treatment failure was defined as persistence or worsening of symptoms or signs of disease after 1 month of treatment.

4.4.3 Mortality:

For patients who died during the follow-up period, we specified the cause of death and estimated survival.

5. Statistical study:

Information was collected using Excel (Microsoft, USA)

Statistical analysis was then performed using SPSS software version 22.0 (IBM company; Chicago, Illinois).

We performed a global description of each variable, calculating frequency for qualitative variables and mean, standard deviation and median for quantitative variables.

6. Bibliographic research

We conducted a bibliographic reference search using the Medline, PubMed and ScienceDirect databases. The keywords used were:

In French: brucellose, zoonose, épidémiologie, *Brucella,* spondylodiscite, sacro- iliite.

In English:brucellosis, zoonosis, epidemiology, *Brucella,* spondylodiscitis, sacroiliitis.

Using the system of associated references, we extended our search and collected further bibliographical references.

7. Ethical considerations

Throughout the process, from data collection to discussion, we took great care to preserve anonymity and confidentiality.

We declare the absence of conflicts of interest in this work.

1. Epidemiological study:

Over the 15-year study period, we recorded 113 cases of human brucellosis in all clinical forms. We counted 30 cases of osteoarticular brucellosis, representing 88.23% of cases of focal brucellosis and 26.54% of all brucellosis cases. Spinal location was the most frequent (22 cases of spondylodiscitis, i.e. 73.3% of cases), followed by sacroiliac involvement in 5 cases. There were three cases of peripheral arthritis (Figure 1).

The sex ratio was 1.72, with an average age of 52 [31-78].

Peripheral arthritis

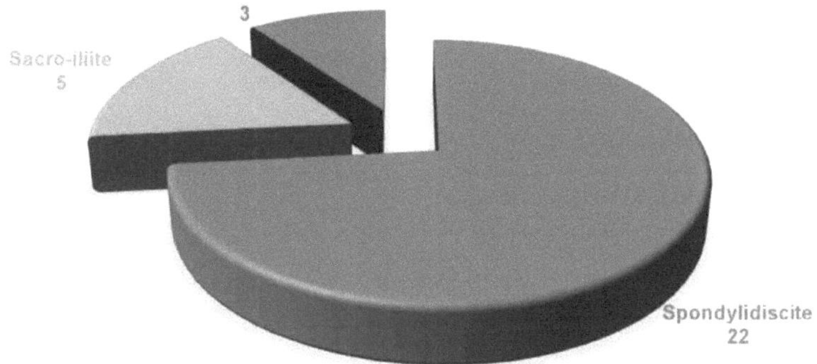

Figure 1: Distribution of patients by type of joint damage

For spondylodiscitis, 13 men and 9 women were involved, giving a sex ratio of 1.44, with an average age of 56 [31-71].

Five patients developed IS. Four were male and one female, with an average age of 35 [18-62].

SI was unilateral in all cases; left in three and right in two.

Three cases of peripheral arthritis were reported. There were 2 men and 1 woman, a sex ratio of 2, with an average age of 28 years [26-31 years].

2. Risk factors for infection:

2.1. Exposed professions

Occupational exposure was noted in 25 patients (22.1%). Farmers and livestock breeders were the professionals most at risk (Table I).

Table I: Occupational distribution of patients treated for human brucellosis

2.2. Contact with livestock, participation in calving and/or milking

Profession	Number	Percentage (%)
Farmer, farm worker	8	32
Breeder and livestock dealer	6	24
Butcher	3	12
Fresh dairy products salesman	2	8
Veterinarian	4	16
Technician in a bacteriology laboratory	2	8
Total	25	100

Contact with livestock was reported by 15 patients. Contact was mainly with goats, followed by sheep and cattle. Among these patients, 7 participated in farrowing and/or milking of the herd without protection. Abortion in the herd was reported by 5 patients. No cases of mastitis in the herd were reported.

2.3. Consumption of raw milk and/or milk derivatives

Consumption of dairy products and/or their unpasteurized derivatives (ricotta, whey, curd) was sought in all patients. It was present in 28 of them.

3. Geographical origin:

Rural or urban origin was sought for all patients. Twenty patients were of rural origin, mainly in north-western Tunisia.

4. Personal and family history

Three patients had a family history of brucellosis: acute brucellosis for one patient and brucellian DBP for two others.

Ten patients had one or more associated defects. These were mainly diabetes (n=8), hypertension (n=9) and dyslipidemia (n=4).

5. Reason for admission

The reason for hospitalization was febrile spinal pain in 17 cases, febrile pygalgia in five cases, febrile arthromyalgia in five cases and finally febrile hip pain in one case.

6. Consultation period

The mean time from symptom onset to hospitalization was 87 days [15-403 days].

7. Length of hospital stay

The average hospital stay was 29 days [1-177 days].

8. Start mode

Onset was gradual in 27 cases (90%) and abrupt in the remainder.

9. Functional signs

All hospitalized patients showed functional signs.

9.1. General signs

Fever was reported by 22 patients (73.3%). Sweating was reported by 18 patients (60%). The main general signs are summarized in Table II.

Table II: Main general signs reported by the 30 patients hospitalized for osteoarticular brucellosis

Symptoms	Number	Percentage (%)
Fever	22	73,33
Sweating	18	60
Arthralgia	15	50
Myalgias	9	30
Asthenia	18	60
Anorexia	22	73,3
Weight loss	25	83,3
Headaches	3	10

9.2. Osteoarticular signs

Twenty patients had spinal pain (90.9%), 52% of which was inflammatory. These spinal pains were predominantly lumbar, in 11 cases. Two patients had gluteal pain.

These osteoarticular pains were associated with sciatica in 7 cases. Sciatica followed the L5 root in 5 cases, S1 in two.

Five patients had lameness. The location of spinal pain is summarized in Table III.

Table III: Location of spinal pain in the 22 patients hospitalized for brucellial spondylodiscitis

Location of spinal pain	Number of patients
Cervical	1
Dorsal	1
Dorso-lumbar	4
Lumbar	11
Lumbosacral	2
Holy	1

All five patients with sacroiliitis had unilateral pyalgia. The two patients with left brucellial coxitis had hip pain, and the patient with brucellial arthritis of the knee had total impotence of the limb concerned.

9.3. Neurological signs

Of the patients with BOA, four had one or more associated neurological signs (Table IV).

Table IV: Neurological signs reported by four of the 30 patients hospitalized for osteoarticular brucellosis

Neurological signs	Number of cases
Motor disorders	
Lower limb motor deficit	2
Sensory disorders	
Limb paresthesia	4
Cervico-brachial neuralgia	1
Sphincter disorders	
Urinary incontinence	1

10. Physical examination

All patients had at least one or more physical signs. Fever was the most frequent abnormality in 16 patients with BOA. Hepatomegaly and splenomegaly were observed in six and five patients respectively. Two patients had associated adenopathy.

10.1. Osteoarticular examination

Pain on percussion of the spinal spinous processes and contracture of the paravertebral muscles were the most frequent osteoarticular examination abnormalities in patients with brucellial DBP (Table V).

Table V: Osteoarticular examination data for 22 patients hospitalized for brucellial spondylodiscitis

Signs of osteoarticular examination	Number of cases
Spinal column pressure pain	14
Pain on spreading maneuver bringing the iliac wings closer together	4
Pain on hip mobilization	4
Contracture of the lumbar paravertebral muscles	11
Contractures of the dorsal paravertebral muscles	1

Osteoarticular examination data for the five patients with sacroiliitis are summarized in Table VI.

Table VI: Osteoarticular examination data for five patients hospitalized for brucellial sacroiliitis

Signs of osteoarticular examination	Number of cases
Pain on iliac wing spreading maneuver	5
Pain on mobilization of the right hip	3
Pain on palpation of the spinous processes in the lumbar spine	1
Local pressure pain in the sacroiliac region	4
Contracture of the lumbar paravertebral muscles	1

Osteoarticular examination of the three patients with peripheral brucellosis arthritis revealed mainly pain on mobilization of the affected joints (Table VII).

Table VII: Osteoarticular examination data for three patients with brucellial peripheral arthritis

Signs of osteoarticular examination	Number of cases
Pain on knee mobilization	1
Pain on hip mobilization	2
Knee joint effusion	1
Pain when moving the hip in and out	2

10.2. Neurological examination

Neurological disorders were observed in three patients: motor disorders in two cases, sensory disorders in one and sphincter disorders in one (Table VIII).

Table VIII: Neurological disorders in three of the 30 patients hospitalized for focal brucellosis

Patient	Trouble editing	Sensory disorders	Sphincter disorders
N°1	Right lower monoparesis	Lower right hypoesthesia	
N°2	Left lower monoparesis		
N°3			Hypotonia of the anal sphincter

11. Biological diagnosis

11.1. Referral laboratory tests

11.1.1. Blood count

A CBC was performed in all cases. Anemia was observed in 14 patients, 9 of whom had normocytic normochromic anemia. The main results of the blood count are summarized in Table IX.

Table IX: Blood count data for 30 patients hospitalized for osteoarticular brucellosis

Anemia	**14**
Normochromic normocytic	9
Microcytic normochrome	1
Microcytic hypochromia	3
Hypochromic normocytic	1
White blood cells	
Leukopenia	2
Hyperleukocytosis	3
Inserts	
Thrombocytopenia	2
Thrombocytosis	2

11.1.2. Biological inflammatory syndrome

The SV was measured in 28 patients. It was accelerated in 26 cases (92.8%) [16128 mm/h]. CRP was measured in 30 patients. It was positive in 22 cases (73.3%) [9-211mg/l].

11.1.3. Other biological abnormalities

Transaminases were requested in all patients. Four patients had hepatic cytolysis. Cytolysis was three times normal in two cases and five times normal in the other two.

Total bilirubin was requested in 23 patients and was elevated in two cases. YGT and PAL were measured in 22 patients. Six patients had elevated YGT and 17 patients had elevated PAL. No patient had an ion disorder or renal failure.

11.2. Diagnosis of certainty

Time to diagnosis, from onset of symptoms to microbiological confirmation, averaged 62 days [4-449 days].

11.2.1. Blood culture

Blood cultures were taken in 13 patients (43.33%): a single blood culture in three cases, two blood cultures in three cases, three blood cultures in six cases and four blood cultures in one case. Five patients were positive for *Brucella* spp.

11.2.2. Serologies

RB was performed in 27 patients and was positive in all cases. SW was performed in 22 patients and was positive in all cases. For the eight patients in whom SW was not performed, three had a positive RB and IFI. The other five patients had positive blood cultures for *Brucella spp.*

IFI was performed in nine patients and was positive in eight cases.

12. Imaging data

12.1. Standard X-rays

Spinal radiography was performed in 26 patients (86.7%) and was pathological in 17 cases (65.38%).

Pinched discs were the most common type of injury, occurring in 11 cases (64.7%). The different types of lesions are summarized in Table X.

Table X: Spine X-ray data for 26 of the 30 patients hospitalized for osteoarticular brucellosis

Radiological signs	Number of cases
Pathological	**17**
Pinched disc	11
Erosion of vertebral plates	3
Osteophytes	1
Subchondral osteocondensation	1
Settling	1
Normal	**9**

Involvement of the lumbar spine was predominant (n=9), followed by the lumbosacral hinge (n=3), then the dorsolumbar (n=3), the dorsal spine (n=1) and finally the cervical spine (n=1) (Table XI).

Table XI: Topographies of disco-vertebral lesions observed on standard radiographs in 17 of the 30 patients hospitalized for osteoarticular brucellosis.

Floor reached	Number of cases
C4-C5	1
D8-D9	1
D12-L1	3
L3-L4	3
L4-L5	**6**
L5-S1	3
Total	**17**

X-rays of the pelvis were taken in five patients. It was pathological in four cases. We observed pinching of the sacroiliac line in two cases, widening of the sacroiliac line in one case and blurring of the sacroiliac line in one case.

Knee X-rays were taken in three of our patients. There were no abnormalities.

12.2. Joint ultrasound

Ultrasonography of the left hip was performed in two patients, revealing significant synovial thickening associated with an intra-articular effusion slide in both.

An ultrasound scan of the knee was performed in a single patient, showing a thin layer of joint effusion.

12.3. Spinal/ pelvic computed tomography

Spinal CT scans were performed in 14 patients (46.6%). It was in favor of SPD in all cases (Table XII).

Table XII: Types of lesions observed on spinal CT scans in 14 of the 30 patients hospitalized for osteoarticular brucellosis

Radiological signs	Number of cases
Pathological	**14**
Pinched disc	7
Erosion/Geodes	14
Spinal cord compression	2
Subchondral osteocondensation	1
Psoas abscess	1
Not made	**16**

The lumbar level was the most affected (9 cases), particularly the L4-L5 level (n=7), followed by the lumbosacral hinge (n=4). Involvement was unifocal in all cases. The topography of disco-vertebral lesions is summarized in Table XIII.

Table XIII: Topographies of disco-vertebral lesions observed on spinal CT scans in 14 of 30 patients hospitalized for osteoarticular brucellosis

Floor reached	Number of cases
D12-L1	1
L3-L4	2
L4-L5	**7**
L5-S1	4
Total	**14**

Left SI was observed in two cases and right SI in three.

12.4. Spinal magnetic resonance imaging

Twenty-two patients underwent spinal MRI and one patient underwent pelvic MRI. Spinal MRI was pathological in all cases.

MRI of the pelvis showed an uncomplicated infectious SI.

The different types of lesions observed on spinal MRI are illustrated in Table XIV.

Table XIV: Different types of lesions observed on spinal MRI

MRI abnormalities	Number of cases
Pathological	**22**
Epiduritis	8
Soft tissue thickening	4
Psoas abscess	1
Spinal cord compression	2
Root compression	1
Spinal erosion	22

MRI confirmed predominant involvement of the lumbar spine (n=12), with predominance of the L4-L5 level (n=8), followed by the lumbosacral hinge (n=4) (Table XV).

Table XV: Topographies of disco-vertebral lesions observed on magnetic resonance imaging in the 22 patients with SPD

Floor reached	Number of cases
C4-C5	1
D8-D9	1
D10-D11	1
D12-L1	3
L3-L4	4
L4-L5	8
L5-S1	4
Total	**22**

13.Treatment

13.1. Antibiotic therapy

All patients received anti-brucella antibiotics. Dual therapy was used in 24 cases, and triple therapy in six. The most frequently prescribed combination therapy was rifampicin and doxycycline (n=20). Triple therapy combined cotrimoxazole with the two classic anti-brucellulosis molecules. The average duration of treatment was 285 days [45-550 days].

Out of thirty patients, five experienced adverse reactions to antibrucella treatment (Table XVI).

Table XVI: Adverse reactions to antibrucellosis treatment in the 30 patients hospitalized for osteoarticular brucellosis

Undesirable effect	Number	Suspected molecule
Clinic		
Vomiting	1	Oral rifampicin + Doxycycline
Epigastralgia	2	Rifampicin oral
Toxidermia	1	Doxycycline
Biology		
Hepatic cytolysis	2	Rifampicin oral

13.2. Corticosteroid therapy

Corticosteroid therapy was indicated in eleven cases. Indications were as follows: epiduritis (n=7), disabling spinal syndrome (n=2), radicular compression (n=1) and spinal cord compression (n=1).

In 8 patients, dexamethasone 0.4 mg/kg/day was used as first-line intravenous treatment, followed by prednisone. In the remaining three patients, prednisone 60 mg/d was used as first-line treatment.

The mean duration of corticosteroid therapy was 66 days [13-180 d].

13.3. Immobilization

Spinal immobilization was indicated in seven cases. Five were immobilized with a plastered corset, one with a lumbar belt and one with a cervical neck brace.

13.4. Surgical treatment

Two patients underwent decompressive laminectomy, and one patient underwent surgical flattening of a psoas abscess.

Surgery was indicated for the case of brucellian coxitis (joint lavage with synovectomy).

13.5. Functional rehabilitation

Five patients received motor-physiotherapy, with four progressing well.

13.6. Anti-tuberculosis treatment

Anti-tuberculosis treatment was combined with anti-brucella therapy in one of our patients. This treatment was prescribed following the discovery of an epithelioid and giganto-cellular granuloma with caseous necrosis on a laminectomy specimen. This surgery was urgently indicated following the discovery of spinal cord compression complicating a dorsolumbar hinge SPD. The patient had a strongly positive RB and SW. It was a brucellosis-tuberculosis association. In addition to anti-brucellosis treatment (taken for 6 months), the patient received quadruple anti-tuberculosis therapy for 2 months, followed by dual therapy for a total of 13 months. Progression was favourable.

14. Evolution

Four patients were lost to follow-up before the end of thoir trcatment. Progression was favorable without sequelae for 20 patients. Five patients were left with sequelae at the end of treatment, and one patient died before the start of treatment.

14.1. Clinical course

Apyrexia was achieved after an average of eight days [3-72 days]. Spinal and buttock pain disappeared progressively after an average of 23 days [6-82days].

14.2. Biological evolution

A control CBC was performed in ten cases. The mean time to normalization was 47 days [9-85 days]. A control VS was performed in seven cases after an average of 75 days [25-185 days] and was normal. A follow-up CRP was performed in 13 cases after an average of 93 days [18-240 days] and was normal.

14.3. Radiological evolution

A control spine X-ray was performed in two cases. It revealed stepped osteophytosis in both cases.

End-of-treatment spinal CT scans were performed in five patients. It revealed erosions of the vertebral endplates in four cases and vertebral osteolysis in one.

14.4. Sequellar remodelling of the right sacroiliac joint in one case.

Spinal MRI at the end of treatment was performed in 15 patients. Of these, nine patients had a normal control MRI and six patients retained signal abnormalities in the affected vertebrae.

14.5. Sequels

Five patients were left with sequelae such as diffuse spinal pain (n=1), spinal pain with sciatica (n=1), radiculalgia (n=2) and gait disorders (n=1).

Discussion

1. Epidemiological data

1.1. Worldwide frequency

Brucellosis is an anthropozoonosis with a worldwide distribution, constituting a real economic and public health problem in certain developing countries. Worldwide, 500,000 new cases are recorded every year(2,17-19).

The incidence of brucellosis varies considerably from region to region. In North America and Western Europe, brucellosis rates are relatively low, with less than 0.1 cases per 100,000 inhabitants. By contrast, in Central and Southern Latin America, as well as in parts of Southeast Europe, rates are more moderate, ranging from 3.5 to 35 cases per 100,000 inhabitants. In parts of Asia and the Middle East, brucellosis is endemic, with estimates exceeding 250 cases per 100,000 population (20,21).

The World Health Organization (WHO) classifies brucellosis as one of the "seven neglected endemic zoonoses", underlining its importance as a disease transmitted from animals to humans (22).

It is important to note that the geographical distribution of brucellosis is constantly evolving, with the emergence of new outbreaks or the re-emergence of the disease. This evolution is due to health, socio-economic and political factors, as well as the increase in international travel. New outbreaks of human brucellosis have been observed, notably in Central Asia, while the situation is rapidly worsening in some Middle Eastern countries(23).

The incidence of human brucellosis varies around the world, with striking figures in some regions. For example, Syria has one of the highest incidence rates, with 1,603.4 cases per 1,000,000 inhabitants, closely followed by Mongolia with 391.0 cases per 1,000,000 inhabitants, and Tajikistan with 211.9 cases per 1,000,000 inhabitants (24).

Moreover, the disease is still present, with varying trends, in both European countries and the USA. Knowledge of this new global map of human brucellosis will enable appropriate intervention by international public health organizations (14,25).

However, human brucellosis remains endemic in specific regions of the Mediterranean basin, the Middle East, West Asia, Africa and Latin America. However, it is important to note that its true incidence is often underestimated (26,27).

In Europe, brucellosis remains endemic in countries such as Greece, Portugal, Spain and Italy, ranging from 0.14 to 0.87 confirmed cases/100,000 inhabitants(28,29). In Greece, for example, rates of 4 (30) and 32 cases (31) per 100,000 person-years respectively have been reported in the western and central zones.

In France, for example, brucellosis is a notifiable disease, and its current incidence is less than 0.1 cases per 100,000 inhabitants, which translates into fewer than 50 cases reported annually to the Institut de Veille Sanitaire(32).

Eight European countries have been officially declared brucellosis-free by the European Union, including the Republic of Cyprus, Estonia, Hungary, Iceland, Latvia, Lithuania, Luxembourg and Malta(14,33).

In the USA, although 100 to 200 cases of human brucellosis are reported each year, the actual incidence is estimated to be 5 to 12 times higher, particularly in counties within 100 km of the Mexican border, where the incidence of the disease is significantly higher (0.18 vs. 0.02)(21).

Brucellosis remains endemic in Central and South American countries such as Mexico, Argentina and Brazil(34-36).

In Asia, countries such as Kyrgyzstan and Azerbaijan record high incidences of brucellosis (37,38).In China, the number of cases has risen considerably over the years, with a peak of 35,816 cases in 2009, almost double the number in 2005(39,40).

In sub-Saharan Africa, although few studies and statistics are available, high incidences have been noted in Niger, Chad, Ethiopia and Tanzania (41-44).

In the Maghreb region, comprising Morocco, Algeria and Tunisia, brucellosis remains a major problem, with animal infection still uncontrolled and, as a result, transmission to humans still occurring all too frequently, despite the various programmatic strategies put in place to combat the disease. The disease is endemic in the region, but has experienced epidemic outbreaks over the last decade. Brucellosis is poorly diagnosed, and the misleading aspects of its polymorphic symptomatology and the inadequacy or non-availability of diagnostic resources are the main reasons for this. In spite of this, more and more cases of brucellosis are being identified as a result of the systematic search for it in a variety of clinical situations, and during screening surveys carried out in at-risk populations and/or those living in the vicinity of a detected outbreak of animal brucellosis. Brucellosis is compulsorily notifiable under health legislation in the Maghreb countries, and is a compensable occupational disease (45).

The World Health Organization (WHO) has stated that the incidence of human brucellosis in Maghreb countries is underestimated by a factor of 10 to 25 (46).

In Morocco, between 2002 and 2019, 314 probable or confirmed cases of human brucellosis were reported (19).

In Algeria, the province of Tébessa recorded a total of 13,670 cases of human brucellosis between 2000 and 2020. The annual incidence rate of the disease ranged from 30.9 (in 2013) to 246.7 (in 2005) per 100,000 inhabitants (2).

Among Brucella species, the most important in terms of risk to humans are *B. melitensis*, which is the most virulent and invasive, followed by *B. suis*, *B. abortus* and finally *B. canis*. These species have the capacity to contaminate humans and cause disease(23,47,48).

1.2. In Tunisia

In Tunisia, human brucellosis is a notifiable disease, and its surveillance is managed by the Direction de la Santé Scolaire et Universitaire (DSSB) under the Ministry of Public Health (49-51).

Prior to 1989, the incidence of brucellosis was low, with an annual average of around 5 cases reported. However, an epidemic broke out in 1991-1992, with over 500 cases reported in the south-western regions. This epidemic was attributed to inadequate preventive measures and the introduction of infected animals from neighboring countries (12).

Over the years, the incidence of human brucellosis in Tunisia has risen, reaching national peaks of 1.28, 2.9, 4.35, 8.94 and 9.8 per 100,000 inhabitants in 2003, 2011, 2015, 2017 and 2018, respectively. The country's south-eastern region, in particular, has an endemic profile, with an incidence peak of 10.4 per 100,000 inhabitants in 2007(52).

A new upsurge in the disease occurred in 2006, with 460 cases reported and, above all, an epidemic in the Greater Tunis region (87 cases)(6,12).

The highest annual incidence peaks were recorded in 2007 (63.6), 2011 (48.9) and 2015 (30.8) per 100,000 inhabitants in the Gafsa district, located in the south-west of the country (46).

The governorate of Gafsa has the highest annual average of reported cases, with 204 cases per year.

According to the latest report from the Direction de la Santé Scolaire et Universitaire (DSSB), the annual average of new cases reported per year between 2011 and 2018 was 551.3 new cases, with a minimum of 140 cases recorded in 2013 and a maximum of 1169 cases in 2017. This variation shows an upward trend in the number of cases over the years(53,54).

The geographical distribution of the total number of cases of human brucellosis shows that the disease has an endemic profile, particularly in the central-western (Gafsa, Kasserine, Gabes, Kairouan) and southern (Gafsa, Kébili, Tozeur, Tataouine) regions. In contrast, the two northern and central governorates (Jendouba and Mahdia) recorded the lowest number of cases, with no more than 10 cases between 2008 and 2017 (53) (Figure 2).

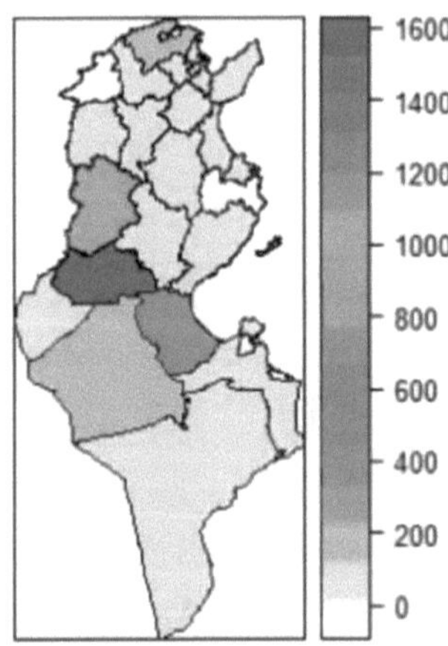

Figure 2: Geographical distribution of the total number of cases of human brucellosis (2008-2017)(53).

In our study, we found a significant increase in brucellosis in urban areas compared with rural areas, with 53 (46.90%) and 60 (53.1%) respectively.

Brucellosis is increasingly affecting urban areas, as in other countries such as Turkey and Uganda. In Tunisia, this trend is partly explained by livestock movements, transhumance and the consumption of contaminated products.

from known outbreaks. It is possible that under-reporting of cases in rural areas, where access to medical consultations and care is more limited, contributes to this observation (55).

In Tunisia, human brucellosis occurs in both rural and urban areas, with rural areas predominating in the past (56).

Human contamination generally results from direct contact with infected animals or their products. In Tunisia, digestive contamination is predominant, which could be attributed to local habits of consuming unpasteurized raw milk and cheese, as well as to certain artisanal manufacturing practices (56).

2. Prevalence of joint damage

In several clinical studies, the prevalence of BOA ranged from 2 to 85%. SI and SPD are among the most frequent complications of BOA [103]. The sacroiliac joints are affected in up to 80% of patients, while spinal involvement occurs in around 54% of affected individuals [11,89].

The incidence of DBP among osteoarticular forms differs between authors and countries, and is higher in older patients [105-108]. The incidence of the disease appears to increase with the duration of brucellosis and in the presence of pre-existing spinal lesions, whether degenerative or trauma-related [35]. In our series, the mean age of patients was 56 years, with extremes ranging from 31 to 71 years, which is in line with data reported in the literature.

3. Type

A male predominance was reported in the majority of series, with a male/female sex ratio of between 1.5 and 5.5 (9,28,57-61).

This is also the case in our series, with a sex ratio of 1.44.

Several factors could explain this observation. It is possible that there is an increased risk of exposure among male staff, given that tasks related to livestock rearing are often delegated to men due to their expertise in this field and their physical ability to perform these activities(62).According to Aloufi and colleagues (2016), the higher prevalence of brucellosis among men compared to women could be partly attributed to the fact that this disease is mainly linked to specific occupations (63).

4. Age

Brucellosis can occur at any age. The overall average age for all types of disease is estimated at between 30 and 54 years in the various literature series. In a Chinese study, for example, the average age was 44 years; in Europe, the average age varies between 25 and 44 years (28,40).

In Tunisia, a study carried out at the Hedi Chaker hospital department in Sfax revealed an average age of between 46 and 51 years(64-66),while in Iran, it ranged from 26 to 46 years(9).

Spinal involvement was mainly confined to elderly subjects, as demonstrated by Koubaa Makram's study, in which the average age for SPD was 51 years (65). In our series, the average age was 56. Sacroiliac involvement is more frequent in younger subjects; in the study by Ariza et al, the average age for SI was 34(68) and in our study it was 35. Peripheral arthritis is also observed in younger subjects; the average age was 30 in Bosilkovski's series (69). In our study, the average age was 28.

In addition, seasonal variations may occur due to climatic factors. For example, in regions where colder temperatures prevail for part of the year, animals may be more confined indoors, which can reduce the risk of brucellosis transmission. On the other hand, during warmer seasons, outdoor activities and contact with animals may increase, thus influencing the incidence of the disease.

5. Contamination mode

Bacteria can enter the human body via the oral, cutaneous, conjunctival or airborne routes (12,32,59,70).

There are two main types of contamination: contamination through direct contact with a contaminated environment, and contamination through food ingestion (71,72).

Contamination by direct contact occurs in three ways: through cutaneous penetration of the bacteria (excoriation), via the digestive mucosa (manuportage) or by airborne or sometimes conjunctival route (a simple projection of bacteria contained in dust can be sufficient to generate an infection) (71,73).

5.1. Occupational percutaneous contamination

In humans, mucocutaneous transmission is possible, since *Brucella* can pass through healthy skin following contact with infected animals, and in particular with abortion products, farrowing products, excreta, soiled bedding and unprotected viscera (74). As a result, certain professions are at risk of brucellosis, such as farmers, livestock breeders, veterinarians, slaughterhouse personnel and laboratory biologists (12,75-77). This makes brucellosis a notifiable occupational disease in some endemic countries, such as Tunisia, Spain and France (78,79). Of the 40 patients with osteoarticular brucellosis in the study by Al Eissa et al. only 33% were infected percutaneously by *Brucella* (80). In the series of 251 patients by Pourbagher et al., thirty-one of those infected (12.4%) had had direct contact with animals (sheep or cattle) (81). Twenty-nine were farmers (11.6%), four laboratory workers (1.6%), and two veterinarians (0.8%). In our series, contact with livestock was reported by 15 patients. Occupational exposure was noted in 25 patients (22.1%). Farmers and livestock breeders were the professionals most at risk.

5.2. Digestive contamination

Contamination through food ingestion is generally caused by consumption of unpasteurized milk, milk-derived products or undercooked meat (22,82-84).

This mode of contamination is common around the Mediterranean basin, in the Middle East and in Asia (85-87). It was found in 55 cases (61%) in the study by Zaks and 79.1% of cases in that of Aktug-Demir(86,88).

Consumption of raw milk and/or its derivatives was found in 28 of our patients. This is probably due to the Tunisian dietary habits of cheese and other unpasteurized dairy products.

5.3. Other modes of contamination

Brucellosis can be transmitted via the respiratory route, through inhalation of litter dust or contaminated aerosols in laboratories or abattoirs (12,89,90). In 1982, in Germany, 15 cases of human contamination by aerosols around the same herd were recorded.

In 1985, 65 people became contaminated during the dissection of two pregnant bovine uteri in a French high school (100% of whom were students in the class)(32,91).

More rarely, humans can become infected via the conjunctival route (by direct contact with contaminated hands or by aerosol)(12,90,92).

Cases of human-to-human transmission are exceptional: sexual, transplacental or post-transfusion(93-95).

The mode of contamination sometimes remains unidentified (96).

6. Monthly distribution of brucellosis cases

There appears to be a well-defined seasonal peak in human brucellosis in the literature, with a period of risk between March and April. This peak coincides with spring and early summer, a period when cow breeding is on the increase, leading to greater milk availability. During this period, cows that have calved during the spring excrete more *Brucella*, increasing the risk of contamination through animal handling. These results are in line with other studies, notably that carried out in Sidi Bel Abbès (97). Furthermore, a study in the wilaya of GUELMA also showed a seasonal peak in the disease, with a risk period between May and April (98). This underlines the importance of taking these seasonal variations into account in brucellosis surveillance and prevention(40,99-101).

Unfortunately, in the context of our study, we were unable to obtain precise information on the exact period of contamination, which would have enabled a comparison with data in the literature.

7. Time to diagnosis

The onset of the disease is often gradual, and clinical signs are non-specific, with the patient seeking medical attention only after several spontaneously resolving episodes of fever(56,89,102). In brucellian DBP, the time to diagnosis was 160 days in the series by O. Jomaa(105). It was 90 days in the series by Koubaa et al (65). In our series, the mean time to diagnosis was 101 days, with extremes ranging from 92 to 227 days.

As for IS, the time to diagnosis was 45 days in the study by Foued Bellazreg (103). In our study, the average time to diagnosis was 58 days for IS.

8. Start mode

In the literature, the mode of onset was often progressive, with a frequency of around 72% (109). In our study, the onset was progressive in all cases.

9. Clinical signs

9.1. Brucellian spondylodiscitis

The onset is often insidious. Spinal pain, often of variable intensity, can start insidiously and generally allow the patient to maintain daily activities, although it can sometimes become intense, leading to complete immobility. In our series, 50% of our patients suffered from lumbar spinal pain (n=11).

This pain syndrome may be associated with radicular irradiation (sciatica or cruralgia), which can lead to functional impotence. In our study, 31.81% of patients had sciatica (n=7).

Physical examination frequently reveals pain on percussion of the spinous processes of the affected vertebrae, as well as contracture of the paravertebral muscles. According to various series of studies, this pain on percussion may be present in 67% to 100% of cases, while muscle contracture varies from 9% to 80% (141).

Patients may also present spinal statics abnormalities, such as a lumbar or cervical antalgic attitude, effacement of the lumbar lordosis or even dorsal kyphosis due to vertebral compression(59,142).

Brucellian spondylodiscitis is characterized by its tendency to be multifocal, with a 10-20% incidence of paravertebral abscesses, particularly in cases of late diagnosis.

Neurological complications resulting from epiduritis are possible, and appear to be more frequent in the cervical region (118,143-145).

The association of spondylodiscitis with hepatosplenomegaly or orchitis is fairly characteristic. It is found in most series (Table XVII). In our series, five patients had an associated visceral location.

Table XVII: Association of spondylodiscitis with viceral involvement

Authors	Country/year	HPM	SPM	Adenopathy
Bosilkovski(69)	Macedonia (2004)	51,5%	30,1%	31,1%
Aktug-Demir(88)	Turkey (2014)	24,6%	14,1%	1,3%
Our series	Tunisia (2023)	13,63%	13,63%	9,09%

Male predominance is a frequent feature of the literature, with a sex ratio of over 2, as mentioned by several authors(142,146). This trend was also observed in our series, although the sex ratio was slightly lower, at 1.44.

However, it is important to note that some studies, such as those by Lopes et al. and Samra et al., have reported a female predominance in certain cases (147,148).

With regard to age, data in the literature indicate that brucellosis spondylodiscitis mainly affects men beyond the fourth decade of life(142,149,150).the incidence of the disease seems to increase with the duration of brucellosis evolution and in the presence of pre-existing spinal lesions, whether degenerative or trauma-related(62).

In our series, the mean age of patients was 56 years, with extremes ranging from 31 to 71 years, which is in line with data reported in the literature.

The lumbar vertebrae, particularly L4-L5, and the lower thoracic vertebrae are the sites most frequently affected by this infection[111,112]. Lumbar spinal pain and sciatic radiculopathy are the most frequent patient complaints. In most cases, only one level of the spine is affected [113]. Unifocal lumbar involvement was predominant in our series (55%).

9.2. Brucellian sacroiliitis

Sacroiliitis is one of the most frequent joint manifestations of brucellosis (151-153). In fact, it accounts for 10-45% of joint manifestations(12,62). It is highly suggestive of this infectious pathology and may occur in the acute or focal phase of the disease. In our series, sacroiliac involvement was noted in five of our patients, i.e. 14.7% of the localized form and 16.66% of the osteoarticular involvement.

Involvement of the sacroiliac joint is frequent, accounting for between a quarter and a half of all osteoarticular brucellosis cases(68,118,135-137,154,155), and was the second most common bone site in our series.

Table XVIII shows the relative frequency of sacroiliitis in osteoarticular brucellosis.

Table XVIII: Frequency of osteoarticular brucellosis in the literature

Authors	Country/Year	Number of brucellosis cases	Osteoarticular location	Sacroiliitis
Aygen(8)	Turkey (1995)	202	94	57(60,6%)
Andriopoulos(57)	Greece (2007)	144	60	9 (6%)
Guler et al(156)	Turkey (2014)	370	108	51 (13,7%)
Our series	Tunisia (2023)	113	30	5(4,42%)

Young adults, especially those aged around 30, are at particular risk of developing sacroiliitis in brucellosis (8,103,136,137). In our study, the average age was 35.

In the literature, a predominance of males has been reported in the majority of series, which is also the case in our series. This male predominance is linked to contagion, which is more frequent in men(9,68).

Sacroiliac involvement usually occurs in the acute phase of the disease. It is almost always unilateral and highly symptomatic from the outset, although it may peak within two to three days(9).Nevertheless, a few studies in the literature have found that bilateral involvement exists, as in the series by Tasova et al. and Cordero-Sanchez et al. who found a high rate of bilateral sacroiliitis in 47% and 60% respectively(157,158).

When unilateral, sacroiliitis is usually right-sided. In our series, all cases were unilateral.

Physical examination reveals pain when the iliac wings are moved apart and together, and when pressure is applied to the gluteal region. Lasègue's sign may be present. Passive mobilization of the hip may also be painful. An analgesic attitude may be seen secondary to lumbar stiffness(68).

In our series, the iliac wing spreading maneuver was painful in five patients, and passive hip mobilization was painful in three. Contracture of the lumbar paravertebral muscles was found in one patient.

9.3. Peripheral brucellosis arthritis

Peripheral arthritis is a complication frequently associated with brucellosis, as shown by several studies(119,136,160,161). Moreover, it is of particular importance because of its diagnostic implications and impact on patients' quality of life(162). It can affect patients of all ages, as previous research has shown(69,113,136).

Arthritis can manifest itself in various forms, including monoarticular, oligoarticular or polyarticular(12,163), accompanied by pain and swelling of the affected area, particularly in the acute phase (154,155,164,165).

According to studies by Tasova et al. and Bosilkovski et al., the frequency of monoarthritis accounts for around 70.6% of cases, while polyarthritis makes up 29.4% of cases, in each of these two series (69, 119).

The incidence of Brucella-induced arthritis varies considerably, ranging from 3% to 77% according to various studies (155,159).

Large joints, such as the knee and hip, are the most frequently affected peripheral joints, although ankles, shoulders, wrists and elbows are also affected, with frequencies of 4.5%, 1.8% and 3.6% respectively in the series by Ibero et al (154).

Other, rarer locations may be affected: sternoclavicular, acromiclavicular(69,154,163), temporomandibular, metacarpophalangeal and interphalangeal(9,119,136,140,161,166-168).In our series, no such lesions were found.

Arthritis usually occurs in the acute phase of the disease, but can also occur during a relapse. Although fever and general signs are common, arthritis may occur in isolation (118). The degree of swelling and joint pain is variable, often intense. Joint effusion is usually detectable. Joint inflammation is often less intense than in pyogenic septic arthritis: significant local redness and warmth are rare. Local complications, such as popliteal cyst rupture, may occur(118).

In our series, two patients presented with a form of brucellial coxitis, while another patient presented with brucellial arthritis of the knee.

Several forms of peripheral arthritis have been described in the literature (Table XIX).

Table XIX: Frequency of peripheral brucellosis arthritis in the literature

	Geyik(163)	Aydin(169)	Bosilkovski(69)
Peripheral arthritis	106	103	119
Knee	23 (21%)	27 (26%)	38 (31,9%)
Shoulder	6 (6%)	31 (31%)	13 (10,9%)
Dowel	8 (7%)	10 (10%)	29 (24,4%)
Hip	61 (58%)	11 (11%)	46 (38,6%)
Elbow	4 (4%)	2 (2%)	6 (5%)
Sternoclavicular joint	2 (2%)	8 (8%)	10 (8,4%)

10. Biological diagnosis

10.1. Non-specific orientation tests

10.1.1. Blood count

Biological indicators of brucellosis are generally non-specific. On the blood count, leukopenia, anemia and thrombocytopenia are typically observed(56,114,207,208). In Crosby's study, anemia was observed in 74% of patients, leukopenia in 45%, neutropenia in 21%, lymphopenia in 63% and thrombocytopenia in 39.5% (209).

Pancytopenia has also been documented in the literature, with prevalence rates ranging from 4.5% to 29% (209).

10.1.2. Sedimentation rate and C-reactive protein

The biological inflammatory syndrome is moderate to frank, with an increase in serum C-reactive protein (CRP) and SV(89,208,210).

Increased SV is common, although not systematic, and remains normal or slightly elevated in a small percentage of patients. Especially in the advanced stages of localized disease, such as brucellial spondylodiscitis, the SV may remain within normal limits(118).

10.2. Bacteriological diagnosis

The confirmatory diagnosis of brucellosis is based on the successful culture of *Brucella* (89,110). Serology is mainly used when culture is unsuccessful or has not been performed. However, it should be noted that serology presents a major challenge in terms of specificity, due to the frequency of false positives caused by serological cross-reactions. On the other hand, gene amplification techniques are of definite interest, although they have limited sensitivity, particularly in cases where culture fails(89).

10.2.1. Blood cultures

Isolation of Brucella in culture remains the method of choice for categorical confirmation of a case of brucellosis. If brucellosis is suspected, it is essential to inform the laboratory of the need to culture pathological samples, as the bacterium has certain specific requirements. These requirements include the use of blood-enriched culture media, maintenance of an optimum temperature of 34 to 37°C, creation of an enriched atmosphere with 10% CO2 for *B. abortus*, and prolongation of culture incubation times(12,89,223).

Brucella cultures must be handled in a level 3 biosafety laboratory, due to the high risk of contamination for laboratory staff(89).

The sensitivity of blood cultures varies according to the phase of brucellosis. It reaches high levels (70-80%) during the acute phase of the disease, particularly in cases of septicemia. However, this sensitivity falls considerably (20-45%) in localized forms of the disease, and the culture rarely becomes positive in the chronic stage. It is imperative to perform the culture within 15 days of the onset of clinical symptoms to maximize the chances of positivity(89,224-226).

Beyond this initial period, the sensitivity of culture decreases significantly, especially if the patient has already been treated with antibiotics, as noted by Sabri in 2018 [202]. PCR (polymerase chain reaction) is a possible alternative, although it is not systematically available in all laboratories. It is particularly valuable in cases where antibiotics have already been administered, offering superior specificity to serological tests in the acute phase of the disease, as noted by Maurin in 2005 and Sabri in 2018(89,225).

The medical literature shows variations in the percentage of positive blood cultures from one study to another. In the series by Bozgeyik and Turunc (58,227), blood cultures were positive in 41% to 56% of cases of DBP.

It is advisable to perform a minimum of three blood cultures, and even up to six, before starting any antibiotic treatment, to ensure greater diagnostic sensitivity.

In our series, blood cultures were taken from 13 patients and were positive in five.

10.2.2. Search for tweezers in other samples

Samples taken include joint punctures, synovial biopsies and pus aspirates from infected sites such as paravertebral or psoas abscesses... These techniques make it possible to isolate *Brucella* and confirm the diagnosis, even when blood cultures are inconclusive. However, it is essential to note that the sensitivity of these methods may vary according to the stage of the disease and the prior administration of antibiotics. However, it should be noted that the sensitivity of these cultures is generally limited(12,89).

10.2.3. Serological diagnosis

Brucellosis is one of the few bacterial diseases where serology is given priority, due to the difficulties of detecting *Brucella* by blood culture. Ig M appears first, and is detected from 10ème days after the clinical onset of the disease. IgG is then detectable, and the titres of both classes (IgM and IgG) rise together during the acute phase of the disease. IgG levels then become predominant, especially in the later phases of acute infection. In the chronic phase, IgM disappears while IgG persists. It's important to point out, however, that it's not possible to differentiate the phase of disease progression by antibody type, as the kinetics of the different antibody classes are not absolute and vary from one individual to another.

10.2.3.1. Wright's seroagglutination

SAW (Wright Sero-Agglutination) was the first serological method described, and remains the most commonly used in clinical practice. It is also recommended by the WHO for its standardization(89). This technique detects Ig G and Ig M antibodies to *Brucella*. Results become positive early, on average around 12ème days after the onset of symptoms (generally between 7 and 15 days), and then these antibodies tend to diminish rapidly in the event of recovery. A minimum significant titre is generally defined as 1/80 (corresponding to 100 international units)(12,89). SAW is a reliable method for diagnosing acute brucellosis, but its positivity may be inconsistent in cases of focal subacute brucellosis (223,232). Furthermore, in some individuals, the presence of inhibitory antibodies may lead to false-negative results.

In our series, SW was performed and was positive in all cases.

10.2.3.2. Bengal Rose test

A rapid agglutination reaction, easy to demonstrate. Highly sensitive and highly specific. It detects mainly IgG-type antibodies, which means that it may give positive results slightly later than Wright's serodiagnostic test, but remains positive for a longer period(12).

A positive result is generally considered to be above 25 IU/mL. Because of its specificity, sensitivity and simplicity, this test is widely used in epidemiological surveys as an effective screening tool. However, for a positive diagnosis or for brucellosis surveillance, it is recommended to confirm results with other complementary tests(89,208,234,235).

In numerous studies, brucellosis serology (EAT and/or SAW) is positive in 100% of cases of osteoarticular brucellosis(58,132,236).

In our study, RB was performed on all patients and was positive in all cases.

10.2.3.3. Indirect immunofluorescence

The advantage of this method is that it identifies the various immunoglobulin classes. IFI identifies the various antibody classes, IgM, IgG and IgA, and is highly sensitive and specific (215,237).

It becomes positive about ten days after SAW, reaches very high levels and remains positive for several years. It can therefore be very useful for chronic screening of the disease(109,238).

In chronic brucellosis, IFI frequently yields a positivity equal to or greater than 80, with complete negativity being the exception (around 15% of cases)(239).

10.2.3.4. The complement fixation reaction

The complement fixation reaction, which is difficult to perform and not very sensitive, has now been abandoned in favor of indirect immunofluorescence-based antibody detection techniques(240).

The ELISA technique is highly sensitive and specific, but the wide range of antigens used limits its standardization and marketability(241).

This technique was not used in our study.

10.2.3.5. Gene amplification techniques

This technique is particularly useful when the prior administration of antibiotics prevents Brucella isolation. This technique enables faster diagnosis (within 24 hours) than blood cultures during the acute phase of sepsis, by detecting Brucella DNA in blood or serum (244).

In our series, we did not use this technique.

For cases of localized brucellosis, detection of Brucella DNA from pus or various biopsy samples is more sensitive than culture. Most tests currently available are genus-specific and cannot determine the species involved (12,215,237).

This technique was not used in our study.

11. Imaging

11.1. Imaging in osteoarticular brucellosis

11.1.1. Standard radiography

Imaging plays an essential role in the diagnosis of osteoarticular brucellosis. Standard radiography is often the initial examination carried out when brucellosis is suspected.

The average delay between the onset of symptoms and the first X-ray is around 2 to 5 months.

The standard radiograph, frequently prescribed first, includes front and side views centred on the painful area. However, it should be noted that this initial radiograph is often inconclusive in the early stages of infection, due to the time lag between the onset of clinical symptoms and the appearance of radiological signs. Indeed, bone destruction must reach at least 35% to 40% before it is detectable on radiographs (57,123,245,246).

The characteristic bone destruction only appears after a delay of 2 to 3 weeks, or even several months. Consequently, an initial standard radiograph showing a normal appearance does not rule out the diagnosis of infectious spondylodiscitis. Disc impingement, an early and constant sign, is detected in 90-100% of cases in many clinical series. In the early stages, disc impingement is often anterolateral, with subsequent progression to global involvement. Its detection requires comparative measurement with adjacent discs(55,247,248).

Destructive lesions of the vertebral endplates occur after the onset of disc impingement, or may be concomitant with it. Initially, this destruction is discreet, manifesting itself as simple demineralization and a blurred appearance. Occasionally, it evolves into full-blown nibbling involving two adjacent vertebral endplates. This observation was corroborated by the results of two Tunisian series conducted by Gueddiche Fatma and Hamza F(215,237),this radiological presentation was observed in 22.9% and 45.71% of cases, respectively. In our study, spinal radiographs were taken in 26 patients (86.66%), and were pathological in 18 cases (69.23%).

Early signs of reconstruction can be seen in the form of osteophytes.

In the case of SI, radiological detection takes around 3 to 4 weeks. The changes observed are comparable to those of other infectious sacroiliitis(109,240). In the early stages, widening of the joint space is perceptible, with blurred, irregular contours and the appearance of nibbling of the joint margins. In more advanced stages, the joint space appears enlarged, accompanied by a loss of periarticular bone density, which reinforces the impression of widening(118). Joint margins become irregular, sometimes creating a "postage stamp" configuration(109,163,249). These abnormalities may be segmental, affecting only part of the joint. Erosions may also be present, mainly on the lower part of the iliac joint and sometimes on the sacral fin. Gradually, a bony condensation develops along the edges of the sacroiliac joint. Although rarely reported, bone sequestration can sometimes be observed(109).

In a series of 9 cases of brucellial sacroiliitis, Gueddiche F noted normal radiographs in three cases (42.85%), pinching of the sacroiliac line in two cases (50%), widening of the sacroiliac line in one case (25%) and blurring of the sacroiliac line in one case (25%).

In a series of 63 cases of brucellial sacroiliitis, J Ariza and colleagues(68) noted normal radiographs in 13 cases (20.6%), imprecise margin contours in 42 cases (67.7%), widening of the interline in 20 cases (31.7%), erosions in ten cases (15.9%), narrowing of the interline in eight cases (12.7%), and bone densification in two cases.

In the case of peripheral arthritis, more specifically coxofemoral arthritis, radiological manifestations only become apparent at the end of the first month. The first sign observed is demineralization, affecting the femoral head and/or acetabulum. This demineralization may be homogeneous or microgeodic, and may extend as far as the femoral neck. Towards the end of the second month, partial irregularities of the bone contours become visible, sometimes accompanied by true erosions, mainly localized on the acetabulum(109,215,237).

11.1.2. Computed tomography

Computed tomography (CT) offers better visualization of the vertebral endplates, enabling early detection of still inconspicuous erosions (250). It is particularly useful for diagnosing infections in the lumbar region, demonstrating a reduction in disc density, often associated with bone lesions. CT also offers the advantage of mapping lesions with great precision. It enables detailed exploration of soft tissue involvement, whether diffuse or peripheral. In addition to visualizing bone lesions, CT is effective in detecting and characterizing any paravertebral soft-tissue abscesses, such as psoas abscesses. This ability to provide detailed mapping of lesions and explore surrounding tissues makes CT an essential tool for assessing the extent of infection and planning appropriate management(251,252).

However, the information provided by CT scans varies according to the region examined. In the lumbar region, it is essential for positive diagnosis and evaluation of bone lesions and paravertebral abscesses. At dorsal level, it reveals details unobservable on standard radiographs, notably gaseous images in bony lesions, and facilitates disco-vertebral punctures. Finally, at cervical level, it helps determine the exact extent of infection(215,249).

In summary, CT plays a crucial role in the early diagnosis of brucellosis-related spinal involvement, particularly at the lumbar level, and guides interventional procedures, while offering valuable information on the spread of infections and paravertebral abscesses.

CT can also be used to assess sacroiliac damage. It can show signs of inflammation, demineralization or erosion of the sacroiliac joints. It can help differentiate the inflammatory lesions of brucellian sacroiliitis from other causes of sacroiliitis, such as ankylosing spondylitis. It allows more detailed visualization of the pelvic region than standard radiography(228,252,253).

Nevertheless, its effectiveness in investigating epidural damage and its neurological impact, as well as in monitoring during treatment, is less significant than that of MRI (251,254).

In a series of 19 SI cases by Hanen Abid, CT scans in 13 cases showed soft-tissue abscesses in 8 (61.53%) and bone sequestration in 2 (15.38%)(255).

In our series, spinal CT scans were performed in 15 patients (50%). It was pathological in 11 cases (73.33%).

The most frequent abnormalities were: pinched disc (n=9), erosions/geodes (n=4), osteolysis (n=1), condensation of the vertebral endplates(n=1) and a psoas abscess(n=1).

11.1.3. Magnetic resonance imaging

Spinal MRI is the preferred examination for diagnosing spondylodiscitis. After standard X-rays, it is the first imaging approach recommended in cases of suspected SPD (256). It allows exploration of the entire spinal column, offering the possibility of early detection of signal alterations in vertebral bodies or discs, as well as the presence of paravertebral, epidural or intradiscal collections (257,258), and enables assessment of the risk of spinal cord compression. It is the most sensitive (96%) and specific (93%) examination for this pathology(259-261).

For infectious sacroiliitis, MRI is the diagnostic test of choice (262,263). It reveals a decrease in T1 signal and an increase in T2 signal in the sacroiliac joint, subchondral bone, sacrum, iliac bone and psoas muscle(228,264).

Fourteen patients underwent spinal MRI and four underwent pelvic MRI. MRI was pathological in 12 cases (66.66%), associated with uncomplicated infectious IS in two cases.

12. Treatment

12.1. Antibiotic therapy

The curative treatment of brucellosis is mainly based on antibiotic therapy, aimed at curing the disease and preventing complications and relapses(12). It is well established that the use of antibiotic monotherapy and/or a short duration of treatment is associated with a high rate of therapeutic failure or relapse on discontinuation of treatment. This has recently been confirmed, notably for the use of third-generation cephalosporins or fluoroquinolones as monotherapy (56,274,275-277).

The protocol recommended by the WHO, and also adopted by Tunisia, consists of dual therapy with different molecules and durations depending on the location of the disease(12,89,279). Treatment of brucellosis is generally based on a combination of two antibiotics active against intracellularly multiplying bacteria and effective in acidic environments(280,281). This combination of antibiotics is recommended to reduce the risk of relapse, which can be as high as 40% when a single antibiotic is prescribed (15,282).

Antibiotic therapy is the mainstay of treatment for Brucella-induced osteoarticular disease. *Brucella*'s ability to multiply in macrophages, as well as the anatomical location of most bone foci, necessitates the use of antibiotics with excellent capacity for diffusion into cells and tissues(278).

Osteoarticular involvement is a common and severe manifestation of brucellosis. Nevertheless, controversy persists as to the appropriate therapeutic regimen and optimal duration of treatment(297).

According to WHO recommendations, the treatment of osteoarticular involvement in brucellosis is similar to that of the acute, uncomplicated form. The recommended protocol includes a combination of rifampicin at a dose of 15mg/mg/kg/d and doxycycline at a dose of 200 mg/day administered twice daily, for a minimum duration of six weeks (118,215,237). This treatment had a similar relapse rate (5%) to that observed with another protocol, combining doxycycline with streptomycin, but with better efficacy of the doxycycline-streptomycin combination, particularly in cases of spondylodiscitis(118,298). It should be noted that rifampicin, as a potent enzyme inducer, considerably reduces residual serum levels of doxycycline, which may explain the lower efficacy of this combination(12). However, it is important to note that the doxycycline-streptomycin combination has disadvantages such as ototoxicity, nephrotoxicity and intramuscular administration(278).

New combinations have also been suggested, including doxycycline and gentamicin at a dosage of 5 mg/kg/day in a single daily injection for 7 to 10 days as an alternative to streptomycin. However, gentamicin use is associated with an average failure rate of 5.2%, rising to 10.8%, while the relapse rate for streptomycin ranges from 2.4% to 12.3% (299,300).

Quinolones have excellent potential for the treatment of bone and soft tissue infections, due to their ability to penetrate and achieve increased concentration in these tissues [49-53]. In the treatment of spondyloarthritis attributed to brucellosis, quinolones can reduce the duration of treatment, the number of antibiotics used, resulting in increased efficacy, a reduced percentage of residual disability, less need for surgical intervention, better patient adherence to the treatment program and a lower percentage of adverse events. Although treatment with doxycycline and ciprofloxacin is significantly more expensive than traditional regimens, it can be economically viable when the need to extend the duration of other treatments, the economic impact of residual lesions and the economic consequences are taken into account. Thus, the combination of doxycycline and ciprofloxacin may make good public health sense(290-293).

The duration of treatment may be extended to three or six months depending on patient response, possible recurrence of disease, and the evolution of radiographic or CT findings (298,306-308). It is important to note, however, that the duration of treatment with streptomycin is generally reduced due to its toxicity. In the case of spondylodiscitis with severe lumbar vertebral damage, a treatment duration of six months may be justified(278).

Recent meta-analyses have shown that treatment protocols lasting more than 3 months offer greater benefits than those lasting 6 weeks (14).

In our study, all patients received anti-brucellulosis antibiotic therapy. Dual therapy was used in 24 cases, and triple therapy in six. The most frequently prescribed combination therapy was rifampicin and doxycycline (n=20). The average duration of treatment was 285 days [45-550 days].

12.2. Corticosteroid therapy

The indications for corticosteroid therapy are specific and limited, but there is some controversy among authors. In general, the main indications in the osteoarticular form are: treatment of acute myelopathy(310) secondary to compressive brucellial spondylodiscitis, epiduritis and neurological involvement(260). However, some authors consider that it may promote dissemination in cases of localized brucellosis(215,237).

In our series, it was prescribed in nine cases (30%). Indications were as follows: epiduritis (n=5), disabling spinal syndrome (n=2) and spinal cord compression (n=2).

In 6 patients, dexamethasone 0.4 mg/kg/day was used as first-line intravenous treatment, followed by prednisone. In the remaining three patients, prednisone was used as first-line treatment at a dose of 1 mg/kg/day, with progressive tapering.

The mean duration of corticosteroid therapy was 66 days [13-180 d].

Progression on corticosteroids was favorable in all cases, with disappearance of spinal pain and regression of radiological neurological signs.

12.3. Surgical treatment

Even prolonged antibiotic therapy can sometimes prove insufficient to treat cold abscesses in the osteoarticular system, particularly in the case of vertebral abscesses. In such cases, surgery may be considered, particularly for large paravertebral abscesses that do not respond to medical treatment. Moreover, surgery is imperative in the presence of severe neurological deficits from the outset. In certain situations, it may also be considered when major statics problems are present, which could eventually lead to spinal cord compression (10,74,140,278,311).

Recourse to surgery appears to be more frequent in the case of cervical or thoracic localizations (215,312,313).

In our series, two patients underwent decompressive laminectomy and one patient underwent surgical flattening of a psoas abscess. Surgery was indicated in the case of brucellial monoarthritis (joint lavage + synovectomy).

12.4. Associated treatments

- **Functional rehabilitation and immobilization**

Functional rehabilitation aims to prevent or compensate for the impairments, disabilities and handicaps associated with spondylodiscitis (140,215). It often includes physiotherapy to correct poor posture and prevent muscle atrophy. In addition, the use of plaster cast corsets for lumbar damage and neck braces for cervical damage is recommended in some cases(311,314,315). Continuous traction may also be indicated in cases of coxitis(215,278).

In a Tunisian series, 40% of patients required orthopedic immobilization, including plaster cast corsets, lumbar belts and cervical collars(215).

In our study, spinal immobilization was indicated in 7 cases, and five of our patients benefited from motor physiotherapy.

13. Evolution

Treatment of osteoarticular involvement in brucellosis is generally successful(316).brucellial spondylodiscitis generally has a favorable prognosis, with recovery usually achieved within one to three months, as is the case with IS and brucellial peripheral arthritis(68,215).

However, treatment failures and relapses can occur, and are more frequent in spondylodiscitis (68,317). To prevent these relapses and minimize the risk of sequelae, it is essential to follow an optimal course of antibiotic treatment and, if necessary, to resort to surgery at the appropriate time.

The prognosis for brucellian spondylodiscitis is generally more favorable than for spondylodiscitis of pyogenic origin. However, residual pain may persist for a prolonged period, and sequelae are possible, particularly in cases of late diagnosis and treatment.

Radiologically, early bone reconstruction is usually observed, and complete restoration can sometimes be achieved(68,182).

Sequelae generally observed include residual pain such as radiculalgia, spinal pain, walking difficulties, etc. (215).

Five patients retained sequelae: diffuse spinal pain (n=1), spinal pain with sciatica (n=1), radiculalgia (n=2) and gait disorders (n=1).

14. Prophylaxis

Brucellosis prophylaxis encompasses both human and animal preventive measures, both of which are essential to control transmission of this zoonotic disease(14,344,345). As far as human prophylaxis is concerned, it is vital to inform and raise awareness among populations at risk of brucellosis, particularly agricultural workers, veterinarians and laboratory personnel. The importance of awareness campaigns and training to reduce the risk of brucellosis transmission to humans should also be stressed (346,347).

Human brucellosis prophylaxis, as far as food is concerned, relies mainly on food hygiene practices and the consumption of well-cooked dairy and meat products from healthy animals.

Key points to know about nutrition include:

- Avoid consumption of unpasteurized dairy products
- Cooking meat to the right temperature: Thorough and proper cooking of meat is recommended to eliminate any risk of brucellosis transmission.
- Avoid contact with blood or body fluids of infected animals
- Wash your hands and kitchen utensils regularly: it's crucial to wash your hands thoroughly with soap and hot water. Kitchen utensils used for food preparation must also be washed and disinfected properly.
- Avoidance of food products of dubious origin: In areas where brucellosis is endemic, it is advisable to avoid consumption of food products from uncontrolled sources or informal vendors, as the quality and origin of these products may be uncertain.

- Awareness and education: Individuals must be informed of the potential risks associated with consuming contaminated food and of appropriate food hygiene practices.

Prophylactic vaccination of people exposed to the PI strain of *Brucella abortus* B19 has been abandoned(12,89).

It is important to emphasize that the prevention of food-borne brucellosis relies heavily on the adoption of good food and hygiene practices, as well as the monitoring and control of the food chain, particularly in areas where the disease is endemic. Health authorities and health professionals have a major role to play in raising public awareness and implementing effective preventive measures.

In terms of animal prophylaxis, disease control relies on vaccination of farm animals, particularly cattle (352-354). Vaccination with live attenuated or inactivated vaccines is widely practised in many parts of the world(355).

The best way to prevent, control and eradicate brucellosis is to vaccinate all susceptible animal hosts at risk, and cull positive animals in endemic areas(357-360). Regular screening of infected animals and slaughter of positive cases are also important control measures to prevent the spread of brucellosis in herds(361).

To complement these prophylactic measures, it is also important to set up rigorous epidemiological surveillance to rapidly detect outbreaks of brucellosis in animals and human cases. This surveillance can be carried out by laboratories specialized in brucellosis diagnosis, using state-of-the-art serology and microbiology techniques. The epidemiological data collected helps to guide control interventions, including quarantine of infected animals and increased biosecurity measures on farms.

Finally, it is essential to encourage collaboration between the human and animal health sectors, as well as between national and international health authorities. Such coordination is crucial to the development of effective prophylaxis policies, and to ensuring a rapid response in the event of new outbreaks of brucellosis. International organizations such as the World Health Organization (WHO), the World Organization for Animal Health (OIE) and the Food and Agriculture Organization (FAO) play a key role in promoting such collaboration(349,362-364).

The main obstacles to disease control in livestock include meagre budget allocation, lack of appropriate services for farmers with sick animals, and limited monitoring and surveillance of *B. abortus* disease. In the case of humans, comprehensive education and training programs are absolutely essential to control the disease among vulnerable groups such as small-scale traditional farmers, healthcare providers and veterinarians. In this context, a collaborative approach based on financial investment between government, semi-governmental organizations, private industry and farmers is crucial for effective disease control strategies (365). A combined effort by veterinarians and health professionals is therefore essential to curb the disease(366).

In Tunisia, the brucellosis prophylaxis program is based on several measures designed to control the spread of the disease in animals and protect public health:

- **-Cattle vaccination:** Vaccination of cattle and small ruminants is a key strategy for preventing animal brucellosis in Tunisia. Animals are vaccinated against *Brucella melitensis* and *Brucella abortus*, the two most common *Brucella* species in the country.
- **Screening and slaughter of infected animals:** Tunisian veterinary authorities implement regular screening programs to detect brucellosis in animals. Animals testing positive are usually slaughtered to prevent the spread of the disease. This measure aims to eliminate chronic carriers of Brucella in herds.
- **Awareness-raising and education**
- **Animal movement control:** Strict regulations are in place to control animal movements between regions of the country. This is to prevent the spread of brucellosis from one region to another.
- **Epidemiological surveillance:** Tunisia has an epidemiological surveillance system to monitor the prevalence of brucellosis in animals and humans. This makes it possible to rapidly identify outbreaks of the disease and take appropriate control measures.
- **Veterinary diagnostics**

- **International collaboration:** Tunisia collaborates with international organizations such as the World Organization for Animal Health (OIE) to implement brucellosis control and prevention strategies in line with international standards.

It is important to note that brucellosis is a notifiable disease in Tunisia, meaning that detected cases must be reported to health authorities for appropriate intervention. Combined animal and public health efforts are essential to prevent the spread of brucellosis in Tunisia and protect the health of human and animal populations(372,373).

Conclusions: Human brucellosis, historically known as "Mediterranean undulant fever" or "Malta fever", is an anthropozoonosis caused by coccobacilli of the *Brucella* genus. It is widespread throughout the world, with a marked predominance in Mediterranean regions and developing countries.

In Tunisia, human brucellosis remains endemic. It is a notifiable disease. It represents a significant public health problem, and also has a significant economic impact.

Given the clinical polymorphism of this disease and its often insidious course, diagnostic and therapeutic difficulties are encountered, especially in focal and complicated forms.

The aim of this study was to determine the epidemiological and clinical aspects of osteoarticular brucellosis, as well as its diagnosis and treatment.

Our study is retrospective and concerned cases of osteoarticular brucellosis collected in the infectious diseases department of the Hôpital militaire principal d'instruction de Tunis, over a 15-year period from January 1er 2008 to December 31 2022.

The diagnosis was established on the basis of epidemiological-clinical, biological, radiological and evolutionary arguments. Brucella etiology was confirmed by SW positivity in blood at dilutions greater than or equal to 1/80, or by *Brucella-positive* blood cultures.

During this study period, we recorded 30 cases of osteoarticular brucellosis.

Rural origin was reported by 20 patients. The mean age of patients was 52 years, with extremes ranging from 31 to 78 years. The sex ratio was 1.72. Patients generally presented two main modes of contamination: occupational exposure (22.1%) or infection due to consumption of unpasteurized dairy products (93%).

❖ Osteoarticular involvement predominated, accounting for 85.7% of all focal forms, mainly in the form of DBP (73.3% of cases), followed by IS and peripheral arthritis, diagnosed in five and three cases respectively.

From a clinical point of view, diagnosis was often delayed. Indeed, the average time to diagnosis was 87 days for BOA. The onset of the disease generally followed the classic pattern, characterized by an insidious evolution in most cases (90% of cases).

The frequency of DBP increases with age, the average age of our patients being 56, whereas in the case of SI and peripheral arthritis, it tends to affect younger people, with an average age of 35 and 28 respectively. The clinical picture for SPD was mainly characterized by spinal pain, particularly lumbar (n=11). In the case of SI, it was dominated by pain during the maneuver of moving the iliac wings together or apart. Peripheral arthritis is most frequently manifested by arthralgia in the affected joint. Blood cultures were taken in 13 cases of BOA, and were positive in five. Serological tests are the usual support for etiological diagnosis. RB was performed in 27 patients and was positive in all cases. SW was performed in 22 patients and was positive in all cases. IFI was performed in nine patients and was positive in eight cases.

On standard radiography, disc impingement was the most common finding in SPD. Two of our patients underwent ultrasonography of the left hip, revealing extensive synovial thickening associated with a blade of intra-articular effusion. Ultrasound of the knee was performed in only one patient, showing a thin lamina of joint effusion.

CT is useful in the early stages, showing disc hypodensity.

Spinal CT and MRI of the sacroiliac joint were performed in fourteen and one patient respectively, confirming the diagnosis in all cases. MRI remains the examination of choice for the diagnosis of BOA, showing superiority over CT and other imaging tests for diagnosis and follow-up under treatment.

All patients with active osteoarticular brucellosis received anti-brucellosis antibiotics. Dual therapy was used in 24 cases, and triple therapy in six. The most frequently prescribed combination therapy was rifampicin and doxycycline. The average duration of treatment was 285 days [45-550 days].

Nine of our patients were prescribed corticosteroids. The most frequent indication was epiduritis (n=5).

In addition to anti-brucella treatment (taken for 6 months), one patient received quadruple anti-tuberculosis therapy for 2 months, followed by dual therapy for a total of 13 months. She was co-infected with brucellosis and tuberculosis in her spine.

With regard to surgical interventions, two patients underwent decompressive laminectomy, while another patient had surgical flattening of a psoas abscess. For brucellial coxitis, surgery was required (joint lavage and synovectomy).

Most of our patients (n=25) had a favourable outcome with no sequelae, and five had a favourable outcome with sequelae.

In view of its extreme clinical polymorphism, it is essential to consider brucellosis and precisely determine its form, in order to direct the appropriate complementary examinations to confirm the diagnosis. For osteoarticular localization, serology is of paramount importance, as blood cultures are rarely positive.

The severity of brucellosis is directly linked to focal forms, which can compromise functional prognosis, as in the case of BOA.

In reality, the best approach to combating human brucellosis lies in preventing animal brucellosis by vaccinating livestock and educating those involved in the production and distribution of dairy products. Applying these measures, in conjunction with compulsory declaration, is the only way to eradicate brucellosis. However, this is no easy task, given its multiple social and economic implications. This is why international collaboration involving organizations such as the WHO and the Food and Agriculture Organization (FAO), as well as neighboring countries where brucellosis is endemic, is essential. A national, multicentric or even international study involving the Maghreb region would be of great interest in order to codify and standardize preventive and therapeutic measures for brucellosis, and thus limit its spread.

References

1. Ramin B, MacPherson P. Human brucellosis. BMJ [Internet]. 10 Sep 2010 [cited 25 Jan 2023];341(Sep10 1):c4545-c4545. Available from: https://www.bmj.com/lookup/doi/10.1136/bmj.c4545

2. Akermi SE, L'Hadj M, Selmane S. Epidemiology and time series analysis of human brucellosis in Tebessa province, Algeria, from 2000 to 2020. J Res Health Sci. March 2, 2022;22(1):e00544.

3. Akhvlediani T, Clark DV, Chubabria G, Zenaishvili O, Hepburn MJ. The changing pattern of human brucellosis: clinical manifestations, epidemiology, and treatment outcomes over three decades in Georgia. BMC InfectiousDiseases [Internet]. 9 Dec 2010 [cited 15 Jan 2023];10(1):346. Available from: https://doi.org/10.1186/1471-2334-10-346

4. Zheng R, Xie S, Lu X, Sun L, Zhou Y, Zhang Y, et al. A Systematic Review and Meta-Analysis of Epidemiology and Clinical Manifestations of Human Brucellosis in China. Biomed Res Int. 2018;2018:5712920.

5. Sannikova IV, Makhinya OV, Maleev VV, Deineka DA, Golub OG, Kovalchuk IV, et al [Brucellosis in the Stavropol Territory: Results of 15-year follow-up of epidemiological and clinical features]. Ter Arkh. 2015;87(11):11-7.

6. Gharbi M. [Brucellosis zoonoses in Tunisia: critical study of sanitary legislation]. La Tunisie médicale. August 1, 2002;80:370-2.

7. Blanc-Gruyelle AL, Lemaire X, Guaguere A, Sotto A, Senneville E, Lavigne JP. A case of atypical brucellosis. Médecine et Maladies Infectieuses [Internet]. 2017 March [cited 2023 Jan 25];47(2):164-6. Available from: https://linkinghub.elsevier.com/retrieve/pii/S0399077X16307818

8. Aygen B, Doganay M, Sümerkan B, Yildiz O, Kayaba§ Ü. Clinical manifestations, complications and treatment of brucellosis: aretrospectiveevaluation of 480 patients. Medicine and Infectious Diseases [Internet]. Sep 1, 2002 [cited Jan 25, 2023];32(9):485-93. Available from: https://www.sciencedirect.com/science/article/pii/S0399077X02004031

9. Hashemi SH, Keramat F, Ranjbar M, Mamani M, Farzam A, Jamal-Omidi S. Osteoarticular complications of brucellosis in Hamedan, an endemic area in the west of Iran. Int J Infect Dis. nov 2007;11(6):496-500.

10. Battikh H, Berriche A, Zayoud R, Ammari L, Abdelmalek R, Kilani B, et al. Clinical and laboratory features of brucellosis in a university hospital in Tunisia.

InfectiousDiseasesNow [Internet]. Sep 1, 2021 [cited Dec 26, 2022];51(6):547-51. Available from:

https://www.sciencedirect.com/science/article/pii/S2666991921000671

11. Doroshenko KG, Rogozenko GF. [Clinical aspects and therapy of acute form of brucellosis associated with opisthorchosis]. Ter Arkh. 1976;48(12):48-52.

12. Chakroun M, Bouzouaia N. LA BRUCELLOSE: UNE ZOONOSE TOUJOURS D'ACTUALITE BRUCELLOSIS: A TOPICAL ZOONOSIS. 1.

13. Akakpo AJ, Têko-Agbo A, Koné P. THE IMPACT OF BRUCELLOSIS ON THE ECONOMY AND PUBLIC HEALTH IN AFRICA. 2009;

14. Pappas G, Papadimitriou P, Akritidis N, Christou L, Tsianos EV. The new global map of human brucellosis. The Lancet Infectious Diseases. Feb 2006;6(2):91-9.

15. Torres AR. Treatment of human brucellosis. Revue d'élevage et de médecine vétérinaire des pays tropicaux [Internet]. 1 Apr 1987 [cited 18 Aug 2023];40(4):373-9. Available from: https://revues.cirad.fr/index.php/REMVT/article/view/8629

16. Morata P, Queipo-Ortuno MI, Reguera JM, Garœ-Ordonez MA, Pichardo C, Colmenero J de D. Posttreatment Follow-Up of Brucellosis by PCR Assay. J Clin Microbiol [Internet]. dec 1999 [cited Aug 18, 2023];37(12):4163-6. Available from: https://www.ncbi.nlm.nih.gov/pmc/articles/PMC85913/

17. Arapovic J, Spicic S, Ostojic M, Duvnjak S, Arapovic M, Nikolic J, et al. Epidemiological, Clinical and Molecular Characterization of Human Brucellosis in Bosnia and Herzegovina - An Ongoing Brucellosis Outbreak. Acta Med Acad. May 2018;47(1):50-60.

18. Harrison ER, Posada R. Brucellosis. Pediatrics In Review [Internet]. Apr 1, 2018 [cited Jan 15, 2023];39(4):222-4. Available from: https://publications.aap.org/pediatricsinreview/article/39/4/222/35149/Brucellos is

19. Nawana TB, Ezzine H, Cherkaoui I, Dahbi Z, Bellefquih AM, Rguig A, et al. Brucellosis at the human-animal-environment interface in Morocco, 2002-2019: descriptive analysis. PAMJ - One Health [Internet]. 16 Dec 2021 [cited 12 Jul 2023];6(13). Available from: https://www.one-health.panafrican-med-journal.com/content/article/6/13/full

20. Munyua P, Osoro E, Hunsperger E, Ngere I, Muturi M, Mwatondo A, et al. High incidence of human brucellosis in a rural Pastoralist community in Kenya, 2015. PLOS Neglected Tropical Diseases [Internet]. 1 Feb 2021 [cited 3 Jul 2023];15(2):e0009049. Available from:

https://journals.plos.org/plosntds/article?id=10.1371/journal.pntd.0009049

21. Dean AS, Crump L, Greter H, Schelling E, Zinsstag J. Global Burden of Human Brucellosis: A Systematic Review of Disease Frequency. PLOS Neglected Tropical Diseases. 25 Oct 2012;6(10):e1865.

22. Chahla B, Firdaws B, Dhrifa O. bouaghi during the last decade.

23. Seleem MN, Boyle SM, Sriranganathan N. Brucellosis: A re-emerging zoonosis. VeterinaryMicrobiology [Internet]. 27 Jan 2010 [cited 5 Jul 2023];140(3):392-8. Available from: https://www.sciencedirect.com/science/article/pii/S0378113509003058

24. Medline ® abstract for reference 10 from "Brucellosis: epidemiology, microbiology, clinical manifestations and diagnosis" - UpToDate [Internet]. [cited Aug 31, 2023]. Available from:

https://www.uptodate.com/contents/brucellosis-epidemiology-microbiology- clinical-manifestations-and-diagnosis/abstract/10

25. Epidemiology [Internet]. [cited 5 Sep 2023]. Available from: https://www.chu-nimes.fr/cnr-brucella/epidemiologie.html

26. Corbel MJ. Brucellosis: an overview. Emerg Infect Dis [Internet]. 1997 [cited 5 Jul 2023];3(2):213-21. Available from: https://www.ncbi.nlm.nih.gov/pmc/articles/PMC2627605/

27. Young EJ. An Overview of Human Brucellosis. ClinicalInfectiousDiseases [Internet]. Aug 1, 1995 [cited Jan 23, 2023];21(2):283-90. Available from: https://academic.oup.com/cid/article-lookup/doi/10.1093/clinids/21.2.283

28. AER_for_2016-brucellosis.pdf [Internet]. [cited August 31, 2023]. Available from: https://www.ecdc.europa.eu/sites/default/files/documents/AER_for_2016-brucellosis.pdf

29. Pelerito A, Cordeiro R, Matos R, Santos MA, Soeiro S, Santos J, et al. Human brucellosis in Portugal-Retrospective analysis ofsuspected clinical cases of infection from 2009 to 2016. PLOS ONE [Internet]. 10 Jul 2017 [cited 31 Aug 2023];12(7):e0179667. Available from: https://journals.plos.org/plosone/article?id=10.1371/journal.pone.0179667

30. Jelastopulu E, Merekoulias G, Alexopoulos EC. Underreporting of communicable diseases in the prefecture of Achaia, western Greece, 1999-2004 - missed opportunities for early intervention. Eurosurveillance [Internet]. May 27, 2010 [cited August 31, 2023];15(21):19579. Available from: https://www.eurosurveillance.org/content/10.2807/ese.15.21.19579-en

31. Minas M, Minas A, Gourgulianis K, Stournara A. Epidemiological and Clinical Aspects of Human Brucellosis in Central Greece.

32. Mailles A, Vaillant V, Maurin M, Garin-Bastuji B. Brucellosis (human) in France in 2006:

33. Georgi E, Walter MC, Pfalzgraf MT, Northoff BH, Holdt LM, Scholz HC, et al. Whole genome sequencing of Brucella melitensis isolated from 57 patients in Germany reveals high diversity in strains from Middle East. PLOS ONE [Internet]. 7 Apr 2017 [cited 5 Jul 2023];12(4):e0175425. Available from: https://journals.plos.org/plosone/article?id=10.1371/journal.pone.0175425

34. Guzman-Hernandez RL, Contreras-Rodrîguez A, Âvila-Calderon ED, Morales-Garci'a MR. Brucelosis: zoonosis de importancia en México. Revistachilena de infectologia [Internet]. dec 2016 [cited 5 Jul 2023];33(6):656-62. Available from: http://www.scielo.cl/scielo.php?script=sci_abstract&pid=S0716-10182016000600007&lng=es&nrm=iso&tlng=es

35. Samartino LE. Brucellosis in Argentina. Veterinary Microbiology [Internet]. 20 Dec 2002 [cited 5 Jul 2023];90(1):71-80. Available from: https://www.sciencedirect.com/science/article/pii/S037811350200247X

36. SciELO - Brazil - Guidelines for the management of human brucellosis in the State of Parana, Brazil Guidelines for the management of human brucellosis in the State of Parana, Brazil [Internet]. [cited 5 Jul 2023]. Available from: https://www.scielo.br/j/rsbmt/a/t9kY3TjkwRCQHfpT5fBZsSG/?lang=en&format=html

37. Çatal B. Rare form of brucellosis, subacromial and subdeltoid bursitis: A case report and literature review. Eklem Hastalik Cerrahisi. Dec 2019;30(3):333-7.

38. Abdullayev R, Kracalik I, Ismayilova R, Ustun N, Talibzade A, Blackburn JK. Analyzing the spatial and temporal distribution of human brucellosis in Azerbaijan (1995 - 2009) using spatial and spatio-temporal statistics. BMC InfectiousDiseases [Internet]. Aug 8, 2012 [cited Jul 5, 2023];12(1):185. Available from: https://doi.org/10.1186/1471-2334-12-185

39. Zhong Z, Yu S, Wang X, Dong S, Xu J, Wang Y, et al. Human brucellosis in the People's Republic of China during 2005-2010. International Journal of InfectiousDiseases [Internet]. 2013 May 1 [cited 2023 Jul 5];17(5):e289-92. Available from: https://www.sciencedirect.com/science/article/pii/S1201971213000519

40. Lai S, Zhou H, Xiong W, Gilbert M, Huang Z, Yu J, et al. Changing Epidemiology of Human Brucellosis, China, 1955-2014. Emerg Infect Dis [Internet]. feb 2017 [cited 15 Jul 2023];23(2):184-94. Available from: https://www.ncbi.nlm.nih.gov/pmc/articles/PMC5324817/

41. Thesis_Boukary_Razac_2013.pdf [Internet]. [cited 12 Jul 2023]. Available from: https://orbi.uliege.be/bitstream/2268/146448/1/Thesis_Boukary_Razac_2013.pd f

42. Schelling E, Diguimbaye C, Daoud S, Nicolet J, Boerlin P, Tanner M, et al. Brucellosis and Q-fever seroprevalences of nomadic pastoralists and their livestock in Chad. Preventive Veterinary Medicine [Internet]. Dec 12 2003 [cited Jul 12 2023];61(4):279-93. Available from: https://www.sciencedirect.com/science/article/pii/S0167587703002174

43. Animut A, Mekonnen Y, Shimelis D, Ephraim E. Febrile illnesses of different etiology among outpatients in four health centers in Northwestern Ethiopia. Jpn J Infect Dis. March 2009;62(2):107-10.

44. Carugati M, Biggs HM, Maze MJ, Stoddard RA, Cash-Goldwasser S, Hertz JT, et al. Incidence of human brucellosis in the Kilimanjaro Region of Tanzania in the periods 2007-2008 and 2012-2014. Transactions ofThe Royal Society of Tropical Medicine and Hygiene [Internet]. 1 March 2018 [cited 3 Jul 2023];112(3):136-43. Available from: https://doi.org/10.1093/trstmh/try033

45. Plommet M, International Centre for Advanced MediterraneanAgronomicStudies, editors. Prevention of brucellosis in the Mediterranean countries: proceedings of the international seminar organized by CIHEAM, CEC, MINAG (Malta), FIS (Malta), Valletta, Malta, 28 - 30 October 1991. Wageningen: Pudoc; 1992. 289 p. (CIHEAM publication).

46. Khamassi Khbou M, Htira S, Harabech K, Benzarti M. First case-control study of zoonotic brucellosis in Gafsa district, Southwest Tunisia. One Health [Internet].

Jun 1, 2018 [cited Jul 12, 2023];5:21-6. Available from:

https://www.sciencedirect.com/science/article/pii/S2352771416300647

47. Corbel MJ, Food and Agriculture Organization of the United Nations, World Health Organization, World Organisation for Animal Health. Brucellosis in humans and animals. 2006 [cited 5 Jul 2023];(WHO/CDS/EPR/2006.7). Available at: https://apps.who.int/iris/handle/10665/43597

48. Kydyshov K, Usenbaev N, Sharshenbekov A, Aitkuluev N, Abdyraev M, Chegirov S, et al. Brucellosis in Humans and Animals in Kyrgyzstan. Microorganisms [Internet]. Jul 2022 [cited 29 Jan 2023];10(7):1293. Available from: https://www.mdpi.com/2076-2607/10/7/1293

49. Medicalcul - Notifiable communicable diseases [Tunisia] ~ Miscellaneous [Internet]. [cited 12 Jul 2023]. Available from: http://medicalcul.free.fr/tn_maldeclobl.html

50. Article medicale Tunisia, Article medicale [Internet]. [cited 29 Jan 2023]. Available from: https://latunisiemedicale.com/article-medicale-tunisie_1828_en

51. Helali W, Bellakhal S, Abassi MI, Abdelaali I, Jomni T, Douggui MH, et al. Brucellosis, a return to the scene in 2017 in Tunisia.

52. Charaa N, Ghrab R, Ben Othman A, Makhlouf M, Ltaief H, Ben Alaya N, et al. Investigation of a human brucellosis outbreak in Douz, Tunisia, 2018. Epidemiol Health. May 18, 2022;44:e2022048.

53. BULLETIN_20.pdf [Internet]. [cited 3 Jan 2023]. Available from: http://cnvz.agrinet.tn/media/k2/attachments/BULLETIN_20.pdf

54. Home - Ministry of Public Health [Internet]. [cited 15 Jul 2023]. Available from: http://www.santetunisie.rns.tn/fr/

55. Makita K, Fèvre EM, Waiswa C, Kaboyo W, Eisler MC, Welburn SC. Spatial epidemiology of hospital-diagnosed brucellosis in Kampala, Uganda. Int J Health Geogr [Internet]. 1 Oct 2011 [cited 18 Jul 2023];10:52. Available from: https://www.ncbi.nlm.nih.gov/pmc/articles/PMC3196682/

56. Zribi M, Ammari L, Masmoudi A, Tiouiri H, Fendri C. Clinical, microbiological and therapeutic aspects of brucellosis: a study of 45 cases. Pathologie Biologie [Internet]. 1 Jul 2009 [cited 17 Jul 2023];57(5):349-52. Available from: https://www.sciencedirect.com/science/article/pii/S0369811408000291

57. Andriopoulos P, Tsironi M, Deftereos S, Aessopos A, Assimakopoulos G. Acute brucellosis: presentation, diagnosis, and treatment of 144 cases. International Journal of InfectiousDiseases [Internet]. 1 Jan 2007 [cited 1 Sep 2023];11(1):52-7. Available from: https://www.ijidonline.com/article/S1201- 9712(06)00034-8/fulltext

58. Bozgeyik Z, Ozdemir H, Demirdag K, Ozden M, Sonmezgoz F, Ozgocmen S. Clinical and MRI findings of brucellar spondylodiscitis. European Journal of Radiology [Internet]. Jul 2008 [cited 1 Sep 2023];67(1):153-8. Available from: https://linkinghub.elsevier.com/retrieve/pii/S0720048X07003348

59. Masson E. EM-Consulte. [cited 1 Sep 2023]. Osteoarticular brucellosis. Available from: https://www.em-consulte.com/article/1411569/la-brucellose- osteoarticulaire

60. Mousa ARM, Elbag KM, Kbogali M, Marafie AA. The Nature of Human Brucellosis in Kuwait: Study of 379 Cases. ClinicalInfectiousDiseases [Internet]. 1 Jan 1988 [cited 1 Sep 2023]; 10(1):211-7. Available from: https://academic.oup.com/cid/article-lookup/doi/10.1093/clinids/10.1.211

61. Nematollahi S, Ayubi E, Karami M, Khazaei S, Shojaeian M, Zamani R, et al. Epidemiological characteristics of human brucellosis in Hamadan Province during 2009-2015: results from the National Notifiable Diseases Surveillance System. International Journal of InfectiousDiseases [Internet]. Aug 1, 2017 [cited Sep 1, 2023];61:56-61. Available from: https://www.ijidonline.com/article/S1201-9712(17)30156-X/fulltext

62. Khelifi C. PROFIL EPIDEMIO-CLINIQUE ET THERAPEUTIQUE DE LA BRUCELLOSE DE L'ADULTE A L'EPH DE OUARGLA (2016-2020) [Internet] [Thesis]. université KASDI Marbah; 2021 [cited 23 Aug 2023]. Available from: http://dspace.univ-ouargla.dz/jspui/handle/123456789/30050

63. Rahamathulla MP. Seroprevalence of Human Brucellosis in Wadi Al Dawaser region of Saudi Arabia. Pak J Med Sci [Internet]. 2019 [cited 5 Oct 2023];35(1):129-35. Available from: https://www.ncbi.nlm.nih.gov/pmc/articles/PMC6408662/

64. Hammami F, Koubaa M, Feki W, Chakroun A, Rekik K, Smaoui F, et al. Tuberculous and Brucellar Spondylodiscitis: Comparative Analysis of Clinical, Laboratory, and Radiological Features. Asian Spine J [Internet]. 18 Nov 2020 [cited 1 Sep 2023];15(6):739-46. Available from: http://www.asianspinejournal.org/journal/view.php?doi=10.31616/asj.2020.026 2

65. Koubaa M, Maaloul I, Marrakchi C, Lahiani D, Hammami B, Mnif Z, et al. Spinal brucellosis in South of Tunisia: review of 32 cases. The Spine Journal [Internet]. august 2014 [cited 1 Sep 2023];14(8):1538-44. Available from: https://linkinghub.elsevier.com/retrieve/pii/S1529943013015672

66. Kefi A, Abid R, Sayhi S, Boussetta N, Battikh R, Louzir B, et al. Brucellosis: clinical manifestations, diagnosis and treatment. La Revue de Médecine Interne [Internet]. 1 Dec 2015 [cited 29 Nov 2022];36:A103. Available from: https://www.sciencedirect.com/science/article/pii/S0248866315006918

67. H. Mahdjoub, A. Benyahia, N. Kalla, R. Ait Hamouda, K.Mokrani, S. Tebbal Infectiology, Infectious Diseases, Batna, Algeria.

68. Ariza J, Pujol M, Valverde J, Nolla JM, Rufî G, Viladrich PF, et al. Brucellar sacroiliitis: findings in 63 episodes and current relevance. Clin Infect Dis. June 1993;16(6):761-5.

69. Bosilkovski M, Krteva L, Caparoska S, Dimzova M. Osteoarticular involvement in brucellosis: study of 196 cases in the Republic of Macedonia. Croat Med J. Dec 2004;45(6):727-33.

70. Laetitia C. Zoonoses in France: assessing the knowledge of physicians and veterinarians.

71. book-epillytrop2022.pdf [Internet]. [cited 7 Sep 2023]. Available from: https://www.infectiologie.com/UserFiles/File/formation/epilly-trop/livre-epillytrop2022.pdf

72. Desenclos JC, Vaillant V, DelarocqueAstagneau E, Campèse C, Che D, Coignard B, et al. Principles of epidemic investigation for public health purposes. Médecine et Maladies Infectieuses [Internet]. Feb 2007 [cited 7 Sep 2023];37(2):77-94. Available from: https://linkinghub.elsevier.com/retrieve/pii/S0399077X06003027

73. Garin-Bastuji B, Delcueillerie F. Human and animal brucellosis in France in 2000. Epidemiological situation - control and eradication programs. Médecine et Maladies Infectieuses. March 1, 2001;31:202-16.

74. Song KJ, Yoon SJ, Lee KB. Cervical Spinal Brucellosis with Epidural Abscess Causing Neurologic Deficit with Negative Serologic Tests. World Neurosurgery[Internet]. Sep 1, 2012 [cited Sep 1, 2023];78(3):375.e15-375.e19. Available from: https://www.sciencedirect.com/science/article/pii/S1878875011016263

75. Rizkalla JM, Alhreish K, Syed IY. Spinal Brucellosis: A Case Report and Review of the Literature. J Orthop Case Rep [Internet]. March 2021 [cited 1 Sep 2023];11(3):1-5. Available from: https://www.ncbi.nlm.nih.gov/pmc/articles/PMC8241257/

76. Breton I, Burucoa C, Grignon B, Fauchere JL, Becq Giraudon B. Laboratory-acquired brucellosis. Médecine et Maladies Infectieuses [Internet]. March 1, 1995 [cited Sep 1, 2023];25(3, Part 2):549-51. Available from: https://www.sciencedirect.com/science/article/pii/S0399077X05807450

77. Zourbas J, David C, Huebner L, Ostemeyer JP. Human brucellosis in Ille-et- Vilaine Epidemiological surveys (1975-1980). Medicine and Infectious Diseases [Internet]. Dec 1 1982 [cited Sep 16 2023];12(12):614-9. Available from: https://www.sciencedirect.com/science/article/pii/S0399077X82800796

78. Eker A, Uzunca i, Tansel O, Birtane M. A patient with brucellar cervical spondylodiscitis complicated by epidural abscess. J Clin Neurosci. March 2011;18(3):428-30.

79. Brucellar arthritis: a study of 39 Peruvian families | Annals of the Rheumatic Diseases [Internet]. [cited 5 Sep 2023]. Available from: https://ard.bmj.com/content/46/7/506

80. al-Eissa YA, Kambal AM, Alrabeeah AA, Abdullah AM, al-Jurayyan NA, al-Jishi NM. Osteoarticular brucellosis in children. Ann Rheum Dis [Internet]. nov 1990 [cited 5 Sep 2023];49(11):896-900. Available from: https://www.ncbi.nlm.nih.gov/pmc/articles/PMC1004258/

81. Pourbagher A, Pourbagher MA, Savas L, Turunc T, Demiroglu YZ, Erol I, et al. Epidemiologic, clinical, and imaging findings in brucellosis patients with osteoarticular involvement. AJR Am J Roentgenol. Oct 2006;187(4):873-80.

82. Human and animal brucellosis: Literature review Brucelose humana e animal: Revisao de literatura [Internet]. [cited 7 Sep 2023]. Available from: https://scholar.googleusercontent.com/scholar?q=cache:bNcZ6fRq8KcJ:scholar.google.com/+brucellose+contamination+digestive&hl=en&as_sdt=0,5&as_ylo=2,023

83. Li S, Liu Y, Wang Y, Wang M, Liu C, Wang Y. Rapid Detection of Brucella spp. and Elimination of Carryover Using Multiple Cross Displacement Amplification Coupled With Nanoparticles-Based Lateral Flow Biosensor. Front Cell Infect Microbiol. 2019;9:78.

84. Lopez-Santiago R, Sanchez-Argaez AB, De Alba-Nunez LG, Baltierra-Uribe SL, Moreno-Lafont MC. Immune Response to Mucosal Brucella Infection. Front Immunol. 2019;10:1759.

85. Kambal AM, Mahgoub ES, Jamjoom GA, Chowdhury MN. Brucellosis in Riyadh, Saudi Arabia. A microbiological and clinical study. Trans R Soc Trop Med Hyg. 1983;77(6):820-4.

86. Zaks N, Sukenik S, Alkan M, Flusser D, Neumann L, Buskila D. Musculoskeletal manifestations of brucellosis: a study of 90 cases in Israel. Semin Arthritis Rheum. Oct 1995;25(2):97-102.

87. Gokhale YA, Ambardekar AG, Bhasin A, Patil M, Tillu A, Kamath J. Brucella spondylitis and sacroiliitis in the general population in Mumbai. J Assoc Physicians India. Jul 2003;51:659-66.

88. Aktug-Demir N, Kolgelier S, Ozcimen S, Sumer S, Demir LS, Inkaya AC. Diagnostic clues for spondylitis in acute brucellosis. Saudi Med J. August 2014;35(8):816-20.

89. Maurin M. Brucellosis at the dawn of the 21st century. Medicine and Infectious Diseases. 1 Jan 2005;35(1):6-16.

90. Ruben B, Band JD, Wong P, Colville J. Person-to-person transmission of Brucella melitensis. Lancet. 5 Jan 1991;337(8732):14-5.

91. Jouan M. Prophylaxis of human brucellosis: towards targeted vaccination of wildlife? A case study of ibex in the Bargy massif.

92. Ee W. Brucellosis as a hazard of blood transfusion. British medical journal [Internet]. 1 Jan 1955 [cited 5 Sep 2023];1(4904). Available from: https://pubmed.ncbi.nlm.nih.gov/13209187/

93. H. N, AGGAD H, S. D, Mebrouk K. Seroprevalence of caprine and human brucellosis in the El-Bayadh region. Revue de Microbiologie Sanitaire et Industrielle. June 1, 2014;8:78-88.

94. Djaafri R, Lyazid B, Denia C, Tolba M. Enquête épidémiologique de la brucellose animale et humaine. cas de la région d'Oum El Bouaghi [Internet]. 2022 [cited 5 Sep 2023]; Available from: http://localhost:8080/xmlui/handle/123456789/14474

95. Human to human transmission of Brucella melitensis - PMC [Internet]. [cited 5 Sep 2023]. Available from: https://www.ncbi.nlm.nih.gov/pmc/articles/PMC3327908/

96. Mermut G, Ozgenç O, Avci M, Olut AI, Oktem E, Genç VE, et al. Clinical, diagnostic and therapeutic approaches to complications of brucellosis: an experience of 12 years. Med PrincPract. 2012;21(1):46-50.

97. Tabet-Derraz. EM-Consulte. [cited 5 Oct 2023]. P-02 Étude de la brucellose dans la région de Sidi-Belabbés à partir d'une série hospitalière (2005-2008). Available at: https://www.em-consulte.com/article/219961/p-02-etude-de-la- brucellose-dans-la-region-de-sidi

98. Touaref A, Ahmed Aimen B, Gouri A, Yakhlef A. Study of human brucellosis in Guelma (Algeria): About 51 cases. Feb 1, 2014;88:57-64.

99. Deqiu S, Donglou X, Jiming Y. Epidemiology and control of brucellosis in China. Veterinary Microbiology [Internet]. 20 Dec 2002 [cited 12 Oct 2023];90(1):165-82. Available from: https://www.sciencedirect.com/science/article/pii/S0378113502002523

100. McDermott JJ, Arimi SM. Brucellosis in sub-Saharan Africa: epidemiology, control and impact. Veterinary Microbiology [Internet]. 20 Dec 2002 [cited 12 Oct 2023];90(1):111-34. Available from: https://www.sciencedirect.com/science/article/pii/S0378113502002493

101. Golshani M, Buozari S. A Review of Brucellosis in Iran: Epidemiology, Risk Factors, Diagnosis, Control, and Prevention. Iran Biomed J [Internet]. nov 2017 [cited Oct 12, 2023];21(6):349-59. Available from: https://www.ncbi.nlm.nih.gov/pmc/articles/PMC5572431/

102. Acute brucellosis [Internet]. [cited 7 Sep 2023]. Available from: https://www.chu-nimes.fr/cnr-brucella/brucellose-aigue.html

103. Bellazreg F, Alaya Z, Hattab Z, Lasfar NB, Ben ML, Bouajina E, et al. Infectious sacroiliitis in central Tunisia: retrospective study of 25 cases. Pan Afr Med J [Internet]. 2016 [cited 5 Sep 2023];24. Available from: http://www.panafrican-med-journal.com/content/article/24/3/full/

104. Lebre A, Velez J, Seixas D, Rabadao E, Oliveira J, Cunha J, et al. EspondilodisciteBrucélica: Casustica dos Ültimos 25 Anos. Acta Médica Portuguesa. March 30, 2014;27:204.

105. Jomaa O, Mahbouba J, Zrour S, Béjia I, Touzi M, Bergaoui N. Spondylodiscitis brucellienne en milieu rhumatologique: à propos de 8 observations. Revue du Rhumatisme [Internet]. 1 Dec 2020 [cited 7 Sep 2023];87:A223. Available from: https://www.sciencedirect.com/science/article/pii/S1169833020305883

106. Dreshaj S, Shala N, Dreshaj G, Ramadani N, Ponosheci A. Clinical Manifestations in 82 Neurobrucellosis Patients from Kosovo. Mater Sociomed. dec 2016;28(6):408-11.

107. BENAMMAR S, GUENIFI W, MISSOUM S, KHERNANE C, DJEDJIG F, BOUKHALFA S, et al. A case of acute renal failure revealing brucellial endocarditis and neurological complications in Batna (Algeria). Med Trop Sante Int [Internet]. 30 March 2022 [cited 7 Sep 2023];2(1):mtsi.v2i1.2022.229. Available from: https://www.ncbi.nlm.nih.gov/pmc/articles/PMC9128418/

108. Jeroudi MO, Halim MA, Harder EJ, Al-Siba'i MB, Ziady G, Mercer EN. Brucella endocarditis. Heart [Internet]. 1987 Sep 1 [cited 2023 May 9];58(3):279-83. Available from: https://heart.bmj.com/lookup/doi/10.1136/hrt.58.3.279

109. Ben Harbi S, Meddeb N. Osteoarticular manifestations of brucellosis: about 11 cases [Internet]. Fac. de médecine. Tunis; 2000 [cited 7 Sep 2023]. Available from: https://www.bibliotheque.nat.tn/BNT/doc/SYRACUSE/1023913/manifestations-osteo-articulaires-de-la-brucellose-a-propos-de-11-cas

110. Guihot A, Bossi philippe P, Bricaire F. Brucellose par bioterrorisme. Presse Med [Internet]. Jan 31, 2004 [cited Sep 19, 2023];33(2):119-22. Available from: https://www.lissa.fr/rep/articles/15026707

111. Sci-Hub | Current aspects of brucellosis | 10.1016/s0248-8663(05)81305-0 [Internet]. [cited 19 Sep 2023]. Available from: https://sci-hub.hkvisa.net/10.1016/s0248-8663(05)81305-0

112. Benkortbi MF, Ould-Metidji S, Ould Rouis B. Study of 8 cases of acute familial brucellosis reported to the Algerian problematic. Medicine and Infectious Diseases [Internet]. 1 Nov 1992 [cited 26 Dec 2022];22(11):937-8. Available from: https://www.sciencedirect.com/science/article/pii/S0399077X05806341

113. Buzgan T, Karahocagil MK, Irmak H, Baran AI, Karsen H, Evirgen O, et al. Clinical manifestations and complications in 1028 cases of brucellosis: a retrospective evaluation and review of the literature. International Journal of InfectiousDiseases [Internet]. June 1, 2010 [cited August 18, 2023];14(6):e469-78. Available from: https://www.ijidonline.com/article/S1201-9712(09)00318- X/fulltext

114. Fethi M. ORGANIZING COMMITTEE.

115. Solera J, Lozano E, Martinez-Alfaro E, Espinosa A, Castillejos ML, Abad L. Brucellar Spondylitis: Review of 35 Cases and Literature Survey. ClinicalInfectiousDiseases [Internet]. 1999 Dec 1 [cited 2023 Sep 19];29(6):1440-9. Available from: https://academic.oup.com/cid/article-lookup/doi/10.1086/313524

116. Cascio A, laria C, Campennî A, Blandino A, Baldari S. Use of sulesomab in the diagnosis of brucellar spondylitis. ClinicalMicrobiology and Infection [Internet]. nov 2004 [cited 19 Sep 2023];10(11):1020-2. Available from: https://linkinghub.elsevier.com/retrieve/pii/S1198743X14637174

117. Al-Rawi ZS, Al-Khateeb N, Khalifa SJ. Brucella arthritisamong Iraqi patients. Br J Rheumatol. Feb 1987;26(1):24-7.

118. Pascual E, Sivera F. Articular manifestations of brucellosis. Revue du Rhumatisme [Internet]. 2006 [cited 19 Sep 2023];73(4):362. Available from: https://www.academia.edu/47590553/Manifestations_articulaires_de_la_brucellose

119. Turan H, Serefhanoglu K, Karadeli E, Togan T, Arslan H. Osteoarticular Involvement among 202 Brucellosis Cases Identified in Central Anatolia Region of Turkey. Intern Med [Internet]. 2011 [cited 30 Apr 2023];50(5):421-8. Available from: http://www.jstage.jst.go.jp/article/internalmedicine/50/5/50_5_421/_article

120. Reguera JM, Alarcon A, Miralles F, Pachon J, Juarez C, Colmenero JD. Brucella endocarditis: clinical, diagnostic, and therapeutic approach. Eur J Clin Microbiol Infect Dis. Nov 2003;22(11):647-50.

121. Lulu AR, Araj GF, Khateeb MI, Mustafa MY, Yusuf AR, Fenech FF. Human brucellosis in Kuwait: a prospective study of 400 cases. Q J Med. Jan 1988;66(249):39-54.

122. Human brucellosis in the Maghreb: Existence of a linked lineage with Europe | PLOS ONE [Internet]. [cited 12 Jul 2023]. Available from: https://journals.plos.org/plosone/article?id=10.1371/journal.pone.0115319

123. Shehabi A, Shakir K, el-Khateeb M, Qubain H, Fararjeh N, Shamat AR. Diagnosis and treatment of 106 cases of human brucellosis. J Infect. Jan 1990;20(1):5-10.

124. Acha PN, Szyfres B, Acha PN. Zoonoses and communicable diseases common to man and animals. Washington, DC: Pan American Health Organization; 2001. (Scientific and technical publication / Pan American Health Organization).

125. Tuon FF, Cerchiari N, Cequinel JC, Droppa EEH, Moreira SDR, Costa TP, et al. Guidelines for the management of human brucellosis in the State of Parana, Brazil. Rev Soc Bras Med Trop [Internet]. august 2017 [cited 19 Sep 2023];50(4):458-64. Available from: http://www.scielo.br/scielo.php?script=sci_arttext&pid=S0037-86822017000400458&lng=en&tlng=en

126. Turki Jaidane E, Ben Chrifa L, Zayani R, Zine El Abiddine A, Abdessaied M, Ben Mansour I, et al. Hepatic brucelloma: about a case. La Revue de Médecine Interne [Internet]. 1 June 2015 [cited 20 August 2023];36:A182. Available from: https://www.sciencedirect.com/science/article/pii/S0248866315003240

127. Yilmaz M, Arslan F, Ba§kan O, Mert A. Splenic abscess due to brucellosis: a case report and a review of the literature. International Journal of InfectiousDiseases [Internet]. 1 March 2014 [cited 16 Sep 2023];20:68-70. Available from: https://www.sciencedirect.com/science/article/pii/S1201971213003731

128. Galinska and Zagorski - 2013 - Brucellosis in humans - etiology, diagnostics, cli.pdf [Internet]. [cited 16 Sep 2023]. Available from: https://www.aaem.pl/pdf-71918-9145?filename=Brucellosis%20in%20humans%20_.pdf

129. Romero Pérez P, Navarro Ibanez V, Amat Cecilia M, Villanueva Garda R. [Brucellarorchiepididymitis in acute brucellosis]. Actas Urol Esp. Apr 1995;19(4):330-2.

130. Alapont Alacreu JM, Gomez Lopez L, Delgado F, Palmero Marti JL, Pacheco Bru JJ, Pontones Moreno JL, et al. Orquiepidimitisporbrucela. Actas UrologicasEspanolas. Jan 2004;28(10):774-6.

131. Hazgui O. 2nd International Military Congress of Tropical and Travel Medicine coupled with the 1st National Congress of the Tunisian Society of Tropical and Travel Medicine and the Journées délocalisées of the French Society of Travel Medicine, Tozeur, Tunisia October 11-13, 2018. Bull Soc Pathol Exot. 28 Oct 2018;111(4):212-52.

132. Mousa ARM, Muhtaseb SA, Almudallal DS, Khodeir SM, Marafie AA. Osteoarticular Complications of Brucellosis: A Study of 169 Cases. Clinical Infectious Diseases. May 1, 1987;9(3):531-43.

133. Unuvar GK, Kilic AU, Doganay M. Current therapeutic strategy in osteoarticular brucellosis. North Clin Istanb. 2019;6(4):415-20.

134. Brucellosis | NEJM [Internet]. [cited 2023 Sep 24]. Available from: https://www.nejm.org/doi/full/10.1056/NEJMra050570

135. Gonzalez-Gay MA, Garaa-Porrua C, Ibanez D, Garc^a-Pa^s MJ. Osteoarticular complications of brucellosis in an Atlantic area of Spain. J Rheumatol. Jan 1999;26(1):141-5.

136. Gotuzzo E, Alarcon GS, Bocanegra TS, Carrillo C, Guerra JC, Rolando I, et al. Articular involvement in human Brucellosis: A retrospective analysis of 304 cases. Seminars in Arthritis and Rheumatism. 1 Nov 1982;12(2):245-55.

137. Rotes-Querol J. Osteo-Articular Sites of Brucellosis. Annals of the Rheumatic Diseases [Internet]. March 1, 1957 [cited Sep 19, 2023];16(1):63-8. Available from: https://ard.bmj.com/lookup/doi/10.1136/ard.16.1.63

138. Gür A, Geyik MF, Dikici B, Nas K, Çevik R, Saraç J, et al. Complications of Brucellosis in Different Age Groups: A Study of 283 Cases in Southeastern Anatolia of Turkey. Yonsei Med J [Internet]. 2003 [cited 3 Jan 2023];44(1):33. Available from: https://eymj.org/DOIx.php?id=10.3349/ymj.2003.44.1.33

139. 05M236.pdf [Internet]. [cited 21 Sep 2023]. Available from: https://bibliosante.ml/bitstream/handle/123456789/7669/05M236.pdf?sequence =1&isAllowed=y

140. Alp E, Doganay M. Current therapeutic strategy in spinal brucellosis. International Journal of InfectiousDiseases [Internet]. nov 2008 [cited 21 Sep 2023];12(6):573-7. Available from: https://linkinghub.elsevier.com/retrieve/pii/S120197120800091X

141. FMS - Theses [Internet]. [cited 21 Sep 2023]. Available from: https://www.medecinesfax.org/fra/catalogue_theses/ville/tunis/

142. Masson E. EM Consulte. [cited 21 sept 2023]. G-14 Clinical aspects of brucellial spondylodiscitis. Aacute; propos de 21 cas. Available from: https://www.em-consulte.com/article/31600/g-14-les-aspects-cliniques-des- spondylodiscites-br

143. Ozgocmen S, Ardicoglu A, Kocakoc E, Kiris A, Ardicoglu O. Paravertebral abscess formation due to brucellosis in a patient with ankylosing spondylitis. Joint Bone Spine [Internet]. 1 Dec 2001 [cited 21 Sep 2023];68(6):521-4. Available from: https://www.sciencedirect.com/science/article/pii/S1297319X01003190

144. Pandit D. Brucella arthritis-an update. Indian Journal of Rheumatology [Internet]. 2011 Mar 1 [cited 2023 Sep 21];6(1, Supplement):75-9. Available from: https://www.sciencedirect.com/science/article/pii/S0973369811600368

145. Esmaeilnejad-Ganji SM, Esmaeilnejad-Ganji SMR. Osteoarticular manifestations of human brucellosis: A review. World J Orthop. Feb 18, 2019;10(2):54-62.

146. Harzallah L, Boudabbous S, Bouajina E, Hamdi I, Amara H, Bakir D, et al. TROP6 Brucellian spondylodiscitis. A propos de 7 observations. Journal de Radiologie [Internet]. 1 Oct 2005 [cited 21 Sep 2023];86(10):1587. Available from: https://www.sciencedirect.com/science/article/pii/S0221036305763915

147. Samra Y, Hertz M, Shaked Y, Zwas S, Altman G. Brucellosis of the spine. A report of 3 cases. J Bone Joint Surg Br. 1982;64(4):429-31.

148. Lopes C, Oliveira J, Malcata L, Pombo V, Da Cunha S, Côrte-Real R, et al [Spinal brucellosis. 4 years of experience]. Acta Med Port. Sept 1992;5(8):419-23.

149. Skaf GS, Domloj NT, Fehlings MG, Bouclaous CH, Sabbagh AS, Kanafani ZA, et al. Pyogenic spondylodiscitis: an overview. J Infect Public Health. 2010;3(1):5-16.

150. Mello CCF de, Souza DU de, Gloria FAC, Moura LO, Mello GCF de. Espondilodiscite por brucelose: relato de caso. Rev Soc Bras Med Trop. August 2007;40:469-72.

151. Neinstein LS, Goldenring J. Brucella Sacroiliitis. Clin Pediatr (Phila) [Internet]. 1983 Sep [cited 2023 Sep 23];22(9):645-8. Disponible sur: http://journals.sagepub.com/doi/10.1177/000992288302200913

152. Ozgül A, Yazicioglu K, Gündüz S, Kalyon TA, Arpacioglu O. Acute brucella sacroiliitis: clinicalfeatures. Clin Rheumatol. 1998;17(6):521-3.

153. Celik N, Laloglu E, Aslan H. Novel markers in predicting Brucella sacroiliitis: The platelet large cell ratio and basal immature reticulocyte fraction. Asian Pacific Journal of Tropical Medicine [Internet]. Jan 2023 [cited 24 Sep 2023];16(1):39. Available from: https://journals.lww.com/aptm/Fulltext/2023/16010/Novel_markers_in_predicting_Brucella_sacroiliitis_.7.aspx

154. Ibero I, Vela P, Pascual E. ARTHRITIS OF SHOULDER AND SPINAL CORD COMPRESSION DUE TO BRUCELLA DISC INFECTION. 36(3).

155. al-Rawi TI, Thewaini AJ, Shawket AR, Ahmed GM. Skeletal brucellosis in Iraqi patients. Annals of the Rheumatic Diseases. 1 Jan 1989;48(1):77-9.

156. Guler S, Kokoglu OF, Ucmak H, Gul M, Ozden S, Ozkan F. Human brucellosis in Turkey: different clinical presentations. J Infect Dev Ctries [Internet]. 2014 May 14 [cited 2023 Sep 23];8(05):581-8. Available from: https://jidc.org/index.php/journal/article/view/24820461

157. Ta§ova Y, Saltoglu N, §ahin G, Aksu HSZ. Osteoarthricular Involvement of Brucellosis in Turkey. ClinicalRheumatology [Internet]. 1999 May 1 [cited 2023 Sep 23];18(3):214-9. Disponible sur: http://link.springer.com/10.1007/s100670050087

158. Cordero-Sanchez M, Alvarez-Ruiz S, Lopez-Ochoa J, Garcia-Talavera JR. SCINTIGRAPHIC EVALUATION OF LUMBOSACRAL PAIN IN BRUCELLOSIS. Arthritis&Rheumatism [Internet]. July 1990 [cited 23 Sep 2023];33(7):1052-5. Available from: https://onlinelibrary.wiley.com/doi/10.1002/art.1780330721

159. Thoma S, Patsiogiannis N, Dempegiotis P, Filiopoulos K. A Report of Two Cases of Brucellar Sacroiliitis Without Systemic Manifestations in Greece. Journal of PediatricOrthopaedics [Internet]. June 2009 [cited 24 Sep 2023];29(4):375. Available from: https://journals.lww.com/pedorthopaedics/abstract/2009/06000/a_report_of_two_cases_of_brucellar_sacroiliitis.11.aspx

160. Rajapakse CNA. Bacterial infections: osteoarticular brucellosis. Baillière'sClinicalRheumatology [Internet]. Feb 1, 1995 [cited Sep 7, 2023];9(1):161-77. Available from: https://www.sciencedirect.com/science/article/pii/S0950357905801530

161. Wong TM, Lou N, Jin W, Leung F, To M, Leung F. Septic arthritis caused by Brucella melitensis in urban Shenzhen, China: a case report. Journal of Medical Case Reports [Internet]. 14 Nov 2014 [cited 26 Sep 2023];8(1):367. Available from: https://doi.org/10.1186/1752-1947-8-367

162. Adetunji SA, Ramirez G, Foster MJ, Arenas-Gamboa AM. A systematic review and meta-analysis of the prevalence of osteoarticular brucellosis. PLOS Neglected Tropical Diseases [Internet]. 18 Jan 2019 [cited 29 Jan 2023];13(1):e0007112. Available from: https://journals.plos.org/plosntds/article?id=10.1371/journal.pntd.0007112

163. Geyik MF, Gür A, Nas K, Cevik R, Saraç J, Dikici B, et al. Musculoskeletal involvement of brucellosis in different age groups: a study of 195 cases. Swiss Med Wkly. Feb 23, 2002;132(7-8):98-105.

164. Kose §, Serin Senger S, Akkoçlu G, Kuzucu L, Ulu Y, Ersan G, et al. Clinical manifestations, complications, and treatment of brucellosis: evaluation of 72 cases. Turk J Med Sci. 2014;44(2):220-3.

165. Khateeb MI, Araj GF, Majeed SA, Lulu AR. Brucella arthritis: a study of 96 cases in Kuwait. Ann Rheum Dis [Internet]. dec 1990 [cited 26 Sep 2023];49(12):994-8. Available from: https://www.ncbi.nlm.nih.gov/pmc/articles/PMC1004295/

166. Bosilkovski M, Kamiloski V, Miskova S, Balalovski D, Kotevska V, Petrovski M. Testicular infection in brucellosis: Report of 34 cases. J MicrobiolImmunol Infect. Feb 2018;51(1):82-7.

167. Scian R, Barrionuevo P, Giambartolomei GH, De Simone EA, Vanzulli SI, Fossati CA, et al. Potential role of fibroblast-like synoviocytes in joint damage induced by Brucella abortus infection through production and induction of matrix metalloproteinases. Infect Immun. Sept 2011;79(9):3619-32.

168. Sisirak M, Hukic M. Osteoarticular complications of brucellosis: The diagnostic value and importance of detection matrix metalloproteinases. Acta Med Acad. 2015;44(1):1-9.

169. Aydin M, Fuat Yapar A, Savas L, Reyhan M, Pourbagher A, Turunc TY, et al. Scintigraphic findings in osteoarticular brucellosis. NuclearMedicine Communications [Internet]. Jul 2005 [cited 27 Sep 2023];26(7):639-47. Disponible sur: https://journals.lww.com/00006231-200507000-00013

170. Ben Hamouda I, Gouider R, Mrabet A. Neurobrucellosis. EMC - Neurologie. 1 Jan 2007;4:1-13.

171. Mehrabi S, Shahriari E, Afrakhteh M, Ranjbar M, Zeinlai M, Haghi Ashtiani B. Neurobrucellosis with Gait disturbance: A Neurological Case Report [Internet]. MEDICINE & PHARMACOLOGY; 2020 Aug [cited 29 Jan 2023]. Available from: https://www.preprints.org/manuscript/202008.0404/v1

172. Malhi AB, Ridal M, Bouchal S, Belahsen MF, El Alami MN. Neurobrucellosis: a curable cause of sensorineural hearing loss not to be ignored. Pan Afr Med J [Internet]. 12 Oct 2015 [cited 13 Jan 2023];22:122. Available from: https://www.ncbi.nlm.nih.gov/pmc/articles/PMC4742043/

173. Guven T, Ugurlu K, Ergonul O, Celikbas AK, Gok SE, Comoglu S, et al. Neurobrucellosis: Clinical and Diagnostic Features. ClinicalInfectiousDiseases [Internet]. May 15, 2013 [cited Sep 27, 2023];56(10):1407-12. Available from: https://academic.oup.com/cid/article-lookup/doi/10.1093/cid/cit072

174. Yetkin MA, Bulut C, Erdinc FS, Oral B, Tulek N. Evaluation of the clinical presentations in neurobrucellosis. International Journal of InfectiousDiseases [Internet]. nov 2006 [cited 27 Sep 2023];10(6):446-52. Available from: https://linkinghub.elsevier.com/retrieve/pii/S1201971206001275

175. Zheng N, Wang W, Zhang JT, Cao Y, Shao L, Jiang JJ, et al. Neurobrucellosis. International Journal of Neuroscience [Internet]. 2018 Jan 2 [cited 2023 Sep 27]; 128(1):55-62. Disponible sur: https://www.tandfonline.com/doi/full/10.1080/00207454.2017.1363747

176. Lubani MM, Dudin KI, Araj GF, Manandhar DS, Rashid FY. Neurobrucellosis in children. Pediatr Infect Dis J. Feb 1989;8(2):79-82.

177. Eren S, Bayam G, Ergonül O, Çelikbaç A, Pazvantoglu O, Baykam N, et al. Cognitive and emotional changes in neurobrucellosis. Journal of Infection [Internet]. 2006 Sep [cited 2023 Sep 27];53(3):184-9. Available from: https://linkinghub.elsevier.com/retrieve/pii/S0163445305003622

178. Akdeniz H, Irmak H, Anlar O, Demiroz AP. Central nervous system brucellosis: presentation, diagnosis and treatment. J Infect. May 1998;36(3):297-301.

179. Masson E. EM-Consulte. [cited 27 Sep 2023]. Neurobrucellosis. Available at: https://www.em-consulte.com/article/1173308/neurobrucellose

180. McLean DR, Russell N, Khan MY. Neurobrucellosis: Clinical and Therapeutic Features. Clinical Infectious Diseases [Internet]. 1992 Oct 1 [cited 2023 Oct 12];15(4):582-90. Available from: https://doi.Org/10.1093/clind/15.4.582

181. Karaoglan I, Namiduru M, Akcali A, Cansel N. Different manifestations of nervous system involvement by neurobrucellosis. Neurosciences Journal [Internet]. 1 Jul 2008 [cited 12 Oct 2023];13(3):283-7. Available from: https://nsj.org.sa/content/13/3/283

182. Ben Hamza Gharbi H. La brucellose: Etude epidemiologique, clinique, et thérapeutique:Apropos de 117cas. PhD thesis; 2009.

183. Shakir RA, Al-Din ASN, Araj GF, Lulu AR, Mousa AR, Saadah MA. CLINICAL CATEGORIES OF NEUROBRUCELLOSIS: A REPORT ON 19 CASES. Brain [Internet]. 1987 [cited 27 Sep 2023];110(1):213-23. Available from: https://academic.oup.com/brain/article-lookup/doi/10.1093/brain/110.1.213

184. Adaletli I, Albayram S, Gurses B, Ozer H, Yilmaz MH, Gulsen F, et al. Vasculopathic Changes in the Cerebral Arterial System with Neurobrucellosis. AJNR Am J Neuroradiol [Internet]. Feb 2006 [cited 27 Sep 2023];27(2):384-6. Available from: https://www.ncbi.nlm.nih.gov/pmc/articles/PMC8148790/

185. Bingol A, Togay-Isikay C. Neurobrucellosis as an exceptional cause of transient ischemic attacks. Eur J Neurol [Internet]. May 2006 [cited 27 Sep 2023];13(5):544-8. Disponible sur: https://onlinelibrary.wiley.com/doi/10.1111/j.1468-1331.2006.01286.x

186. Oueslati I, Berriche A, Ammari L, Abdelmalek R, Kanoun F, Kilani B, et al. Epidemiological and clinical characteristics of neurobrucellosis case patients in Tunisia. Medicine and Infectious Diseases [Internet]. May 2016 [cited 27 Sep 2023];46(3):123-30. Available from: https://linkinghub.elsevier.com/retrieve/pii/S0399077X16000135

187. Ben Khalfallah A, Ousji M, Annabi N, Ajili F, Tlili R. Brucellian endocarditis: clinical features and therapeutic modalities. Annales de Cardiologie et d'Angéiologie [Internet]. June 2006 [cited 6 Apr 2023];55(3):157-60. Available from: https://linkinghub.elsevier.com/retrieve/pii/S0003392805000284

188. Fernandez-Guerrero ML. Zoonotic endocarditis. Infect Dis Clin North Am. March 1993;7(1):135-52.

189. Heibig J, Beall AC, Myers R, Harder E, Feteih N. Brucella aortic endocarditis corrected by prosthetic valve replacement. American Heart Journal [Internet]. 1983 Sep 1 [cited 2023 Sep 28];106(3):594-6. Available from: https://www.sciencedirect.com/science/article/pii/000287038390710X

190. Jacobs F, Abramowicz D, Vereerstraeten P, Le Clerc JL, Zecb F, Thys JP. Brucella Endocarditis: The Role of Combined Medical and Surgical Treatment. Reviews of Infectious Diseases [Internet]. 1990 Sep 1 [cited 2023 Sep 30];12(5):740-4. Available from: https://doi.org/10.1093/clinids/12.5.740

191. Zumla A. Mandell, Douglas, and Bennett's principles and practice of infectious diseases. Lancet Infect Dis [Internet]. May 2010 [cited 30 Sep 2023];10(5):303-4. Available from: https://www.ncbi.nlm.nih.gov/pmc/articles/PMC7128814/

192. Peery TM, Belter LF. Brucellosis and heart disease. II. Fatal brucellosis: a review of the literature and report of new cases. Am J Pathol. June 1960;36(6):673-97.

193. Tripp L, Sawchuk LA. Undulant Fever: Colonialism, Culture, and Compliancy.

194. Ariza J, Corredoira J, Pallares R, Viladrich PF, Rufi G, Pujol M, et al. Characteristics of and Risk Factors for Relapse of Brucellosis in Humans. ClinicalInfectiousDiseases [Internet]. 1995 [cited 28 Sep 2023];20(5):1241-9. Available from: https://www.jstor.org/stable/4458535

195. Spink WesleyW. HOST-PARASITE RELATIONSHIP IN BRUCELLOSIS. The Lancet [Internet]. Jul 1964 [cited 28 Sep 2023];284(7352):161-4. Available from: https://linkinghub.elsevier.com/retrieve/pii/S0140673664902284

196. first-page-pdf.pdf [Internet]. [cited 28 Sep 2023]. Available from: https://www.sciencedirect.com/sdfe/pdf/download/eid/1-s2.0-000287038390710X/first-page-pdf

197. Keshtkar-Jahromi M, Razavi SM, Gholamin S, Keshtkar-Jahromi M, Hossain M, Sajadi M. MEDICAL vs. MEDICAL AND SURGICAL TREATMENT FOR BRUCELLA ENDOCARDITIS: A REVIEW OF THE LITERATURE. Ann Thorac Surg. Dec 2012;94(6):2141-6.

198. Cohen PS, Maguire JH, Weinstein L. Infective endocarditis caused by gram-negative bacteria: A review of the literature, 1945-1977. Progress in CardiovascularDiseases [Internet]. Jan 1980 [cited 28 Sep 2023];22(4):205-42. Available from: https://linkinghub.elsevier.com/retrieve/pii/0033062080900109

199. Taamallah K, Hammami F, Gharsallah H, Koubaa M, Ben Jemaa M, Fehri W. Brucella Prosthetic Valve Endocarditis: A Systematic Review. J SaudiHeart Assoc. 2021;33(3):198-212.

200. Tunisie_Med_2012_90_4_335_336.pdf [Internet]. [cited 28 Sep 2023]. Available from: https://applications.emro.who.int/imemrf/Tunisie_Med/Tunisie_Med_2012_90_4_335_336.pdf

201. Bayer AS, Bolger AF, Taubert KA, Wilson W, Steckelberg J, Karchmer AW, et al. Diagnosis and management of infective endocarditis and its complications. Circulation. Dec 22 1998;98(25):2936-48.

202. Jin M, Fan Z, Gao R, Li X, Gao Z, Wang Z. Research progress on complications of Brucellosis. Front Cell Infect Microbiol. 2023;13:1136674.

203. Tuncer M, Ekim H, Günes Y, Güntekin Ü. Atrial Septal Defect Presenting With Brucella Endocarditis. Circulation Journal. 2008;72(12):2096-7.

204. Sabzi F, Heidari A, Faraji R. Right ventricular outflow tract endocarditis caused by brucellosis. Journal of Infection and Public Health [Internet]. Sep 1, 2017 [cited Sep 30, 2023];10(5):678-80. Available from: https://www.sciencedirect.com/science/article/pii/S1876034116301496

205. Sci-Hub | Brucella endocarditis complicated with a mycotic aneurysm of the superior mesenteric artery: a case report | 10.1016/s0167-5273(03)00166-9 [Internet]. [cited 30 Sep 2023]. Available from: https://sci-hub.hkvisa.net/10.1016/s0167-5273(03)00166-9

206. Altekin RE, Karakas MS, Yanikoglu A, Ozbek SC, Akdemir B, Demirtas H, et al. Aortic valve endocarditis and cerebral mycotic aneurysm due to brucellosis. Journal of Cardiology Cases [Internet]. Dec 1, 2011 [cited Sep 30, 2023];4(3):e179-82. Available from: https://www.journalofcardiologycases.com/article/S1878-5409(11)00058- 2/fulltext

207. Raschilas F, Cordonnier C, Grasland A, Casetta A, Boussougant Y, Pouchot J, et al. Pancytopenia during acute brucellosis. La Revue de Médecine Interne [Internet]. 1 Jan 1997 [cited 30 Sep 2023];18(12):972-4. Available from: https://www.sciencedirect.com/science/article/pii/S0248866397801178

208. Bellamine K, Riyad M, Takourt B, Farouqi B, Fellah H. BIOLOGICAL DIAGNOSIS OF HUMAN BRUCELLOSIS: COMPARISON OF TWO SEROAGGLUTINATION TECHNIQUES. 2012;7.

209. Crosby E, Llosa L, Quesada MM, Carrillo P. C, Gotuzzo E. Hematologic Changes in Brucellosis. The Journal of Infectious Diseases [Internet]. 1984 Sep 1 [cited 2023 Sep 30];150(3):419-24. Available from: https://doi.org/10.1093/infdis/150.3.419

210. Bonaldi V, Padovani B, Chami M, Nectoux F, Grimaud A. [MRI and chronic osteoarticular infections. Contribution of inversion-recovery sequence with fat signal cancellation in the follow-up of chronic osteitis under medical treatment. Apropos of 14 cases. J Radiol. March 1, 1991;72(3):149-55.

211. Navarro JM, Mendoza J, Leiva J, Rodrïguez-Contreras R, De La Rosa M. C-reactive protein as a prognostic indicator in acute brucellosis. Diagnostic Microbiology and Infectious Disease [Internet]. May 1990 [cited 2 Oct 2023];13(3):269-70. Available from: https://linkinghub.elsevier.com/retrieve/pii/0732889390900713

212. Tohmé A, Hammoud A, el Rassi B, Germanos-Haddad M, Ghayad E. [Human brucellosis. Retrospective studies of 63 cases in Lebanon]. Presse Med. 29 sept 2001;30(27):1339-43.

213. Neau D, Bonnet F, Ragnaud JM, Pellegrin JL, Schaeverbeke T, Monlun E, et al. Retrospective study of 59 cases of human brucellosis in Aquitaine. Clinical, biological and therapeutic aspects. Medicine and Infectious Diseases [Internet]. 1 June 1997 [cited 2 Oct 2023];27:638-41. Available from: https://www.sciencedirect.com/science/article/pii/S0399077X97802156

214. Bosilkovski M, Krteva L, Dimzova M, Kondova I. Brucellosis in 418 patients from the Balkan Peninsula: exposure-related differences in clinical manifestations, laboratory test results, and therapy outcome. International Journal of InfectiousDiseases [Internet]. 1 Jul 2007 [cited 2 Oct 2023];11(4):342-7. Available from: https://www.sciencedirect.com/science/article/pii/S1201971206001895

215. Hamza F. OSTERO-ARTICULAR BRUCELLOSIS: EPIDEMIOCLINICAL AND THERAPEUTIC STUDY [Internet]. DOCTOR OF MEDICINE; 2018. Available from: file:///C:/Users/H/Desktop/Faycel%20HAMZA0.pdf.

216. Sci-Hub | Brucella meningitis | 10.1016/s0163-4453(87)91952-9 [Internet]. [cited 3 Oct 2023]. Available from: https://sci-hub.hkvisa.net/10.1016/s0163-4453(87)91952-9

217. Al-Sous MW, Bohlega S, Al-Kawi MZ, Alwatban J, McLean DR. Neurobrucellosis: Clinical and Neuroimaging Correlation. AJNR Am J Neuroradiol [Internet]. 2004 Mar [cited 2023 Oct 3];25(3):395-401. Available from: https://www.ncbi.nlm.nih.gov/pmc/articles/PMC8158553/

218. Sci-Hub | Paediatric neurobrucellosis: case report and literature review | 10.1016/s0163-4453(98)90647-8 [Internet]. [cited 3 Oct 2023]. Disponible sur: https://sci-hub.hkvisa.net/10.1016/s0163-4453(98)90647-8

219. Godfroid J, Kasbohrer A. Brucellosis in the European Union and Norway at the turn of the twenty-first century. Vet Microbiol. 2002 Dec 20;90(1-4):135-45.

220. Challoner KR, Riley KB, Larsen RA. Brucella meningitis. The American Journal of Emergency Medicine [Internet]. Jan 1990 [cited Oct 3, 2023];8(1):40-2. Available from: https://linkinghub.elsevier.com/retrieve/pii/0735675790902939

221. KOUSSA S, TOHME A, GHAYAD E, NASNAS R, EL KALLAB K, CHEMALY R. Neurobrucellosis: clinical and therapeutic studies of 15 patients. Rev neurol (Paris). 2003;159(12):1148-55.

222. Gouider R, Samet S, Triki C, Fredj M, Gargouri A, el Bahri F, et al [Neurological manifestations indicative of brucellosis]. Rev Neurol (Paris). March 1999;155(3):215-8.

223. Roux J. Biological diagnosis of brucellosis in humans. Médecine et Maladies Infectieuses [Internet]. 1 May 1974 [cited 1 Oct 2023];4(5):259-66. Available from: https://www.sciencedirect.com/science/article/pii/S0399077X7480137X

224. Yagupsky P, Morata P, Colmenero JD. Laboratory Diagnosis of Human Brucellosis. Clin Microbiol Rev. Dec 18, 2019;33(1):e00073-19.

225. Nawel MA. Mémoire de Fin d'Etudes Diplôme d'Etudes Supérieures Option: Microbiologie.

226. Ines G, Sana B, Ahlam Z. Epidemiology of brucellosis in the wilaya of Guelma [Internet]. SNV.STU; 2020 [cited 1 Oct 2023]. Available from: http://dspace.univ-guelma.dz/jspui/handle/123456789/10772

227. Turunc T, Ziya Demiroglu Y, Uncu H, Colakoglu S, Arslan H. A comparative analysis of tuberculous, brucellar and pyogenic spontaneous spondylodiscitis patients. Journal of Infection [Internet]. August 2007 [cited 2 Oct 2023];55(2):158-63. Available from: https://linkinghub.elsevier.com/retrieve/pii/S0163445307000953

228. Abid R, Smaoui O, Oueslati I, Hannachi S, Battih R, Louzir B. Neurobrucellosis: An Unusual Location of Brucellosis. Annals of Clinical Case Reports - Internal Medicine [Internet]. [cited 2 Oct 2023];3. Available from: https://www.anncaserep.com/full-text/accr-v3-id1525.php

229. Mancini P, Bottaro V, Capitani F, De Soccio G, Prosperini L, Restaino P, et al. Recurrent Bell's palsy: outcomes and correlation with clinical comorbidities. Acta Otorhinolaryngol Ital. oct 2019;39(5):316-21.

230. Du N, Wang F. Clinical characteristics and outcome of Brucella endocarditis. Turk J Med Sci. Dec 20, 2016;46(6):1729-33.

231. Assya H, HAMOU Assya. Epidemiological survey on brucellosis at the level of the wilaya of Tlemcen and creation of a DNA biothèque for case-control study. tlemcen: bibfac.univ-tlemcen.dz/snvstu; 2016.

232. Ulu-Kilic A, Metan G, Alp E. Clinical presentations and diagnosis of brucellosis. Recent Pat Antiinfect Drug Discov. Apr 2013;8(1): 34-41.

233. BRUCELLA [Internet]. [cited 5 Oct 2023]. Available from: http://www.microbes-edu.org/etudiant/brucella.html

234. Nielsen K. Diagnosis of brucellosis by serology. Veterinary Microbiology [Internet]. 20 Dec 2002 [cited 2 Oct 2023];90(1):447-59. Available from: https://www.sciencedirect.com/science/article/pii/S0378113502002298

235. Samaha H, Mohamed TR, Khoudair RM, Ashour HM. Serodiagnosis of brucellosis in cattle and humans in Egypt. Immunobiology. 2009;214(3):223-6.

236. Hashemi SH, Keramat F, Ranjbar M, Mamani M, Farzam A, Jamal-Omidi S. Osteoarticular complications of brucellosis in Hamedan, an endemic area in the west of Iran. International Journal of InfectiousDiseases. 1 Nov 2007;11(6):496-500.

237. Fatma G. LA BRUCELLOSE: ÉPIDÉMIO CLINIQUE DES CASES HOSPITALISÉS À L'HÔPITAL LA RABTA (2003-2017) [Internet]. DOCTOR OF MEDICINE; 2020. Available from: file:///C:/Users/H/Desktop/THESE%20Fatma%20GUEDDICHE%20FINALE%200. Pdf el-Desouki M. Skeletal brucellosis: assessment with bone scintigraphy.

238. Radiology [Internet]. 1991 Nov [cited 2023 Oct 2];181(2):415-8. Available from: http://pubs.rsna.org/doi/10.1148/radiology.181.2.1924782

239. Pillot J, Kouyoumdjian S, Grangeot L. [Serodiagnosis of human brucellosis]. Nouv Presse Med. 11 Jan 1975;04(2):105-8.

240. Catalogue-Thematique-des-Theses-2021.pdf [Internet]. [cited 3 Oct 2023]. Available from: https://fmt.rnu.tn/wp-content/uploads/2021/11/Catalogue-Thematique-des-Theses-2021.pdf

241. Yu WL, Nielsen K. Review of Detection of Brucella sp. by Polymerase Chain Reaction. Croat Med J [Internet]. August 2010 [cited 3 Oct 2023];51(4):306-13. Available from: https://www.ncbi.nlm.nih.gov/pmc/articles/PMC2931435/

242. Mantecon MÂ, Gutiérrez P, Zarzosa MDP, Duenas AI, Solera J, Fernandez- Lago L, et al. Utility of an immunocapture-agglutination test and an enzyme- linked immunosorbent assay test against cytosolic proteins from Brucella melitensis B115 in the diagnosis and follow-up of human acute brucellosis. Diagnostic Microbiology and InfectiousDisease [Internet]. May 2006 [cited 3 Oct 2023];55(1):27-35. Available from: https://linkinghub.elsevier.com/retrieve/pii/S0732889305003391

243. MARMONIER A, B B. APPLICATION OF THE ELISA (ENZYME-LINKED-IMMUNOSORBENT-ASSAY) IMMUNOENZYMATIC TECHNIQUE TO THE SEROLOGICAL DIAGNOSIS OF HUMAN BRUCELLOSIS. I: EVALUATION OF SOME REACTION PARAMETERS AND PRACTICAL APPLICATION. APPLICATION OF THE ELISA (ENZYME-LINKED-IMMUNOSORBENT-ASSAY) IMMUNOENZYMATIC TECHNIQUE TO THE SEROLOGICAL DIAGNOSIS OF HUMAN BRUCELLOSIS I: EVALUATION OF SOME REACTION PARAMETERS AND PRACTICAL APPLICATION. 1981;

244. Masson E. EM-Consulte. [cited 3 Oct 2023]. Non-tuberculous infectious spondylodiscitis. Available from: https://www.em-consulte.com/article/50928/spondylodiscite-infectious-non-tuberculous.

245. Crump JA, Youssef FG, Luby SP, Wasfy MO, Rangel JM, Taalat M, et al. Estimating the Incidence of Typhoid Fever and Other Febrile Illnesses in Developing Countries. Emerg Infect Dis. May 2003;9(5):539-44.

246. Cash-Goldwasser S, Maze MJ, Rubach MP, Biggs HM, Stoddard RA, Sharples KJ, et al. Risk Factors for Human Brucellosis in Northern Tanzania. Am J Trop Med Hyg. Feb 2018;98(2):598-606.

247. Guerrier G, Daronat JM, Morisse L, Yvon JF, Pappas G. Epidemiological and clinical aspects of human Brucella suis infection in Polynesia. Epidemiol Infect. Oct 2011;139(10):1621-5.

248. Karadzinska-Bislimovska J, Minov J, Mijakoski D, Stoleski S, Todorov S. Brucellosis as an Occupational Disease in the Republic of Macedonia. Macedonian Journal of Medical Sciences [Internet]. 15 Sep 2010 [cited 3 Oct 2023];3(3):251-6. Available from: http://versita.metapress.com/openurl.asp?genre=article&id=doi:10.3889/MJMS.1857-5773.2010.0129

249. Masson E. EM-Consulte. [cited 21 sept 2023]. Osteoarticular manifestations of brucellosis. Available from: https://www.em-consulte.com/article/8233/manifestations-osteoarticulaires-de-la-brucellose

250. Masson E. EM-Consulte. [cited 5 Oct 2023]. Diagnostic imaging of infectious spondylodiscitis. Available from: https://www.em-consulte.com/article/25509/references/imagerie-diagnostique-de-la-spondylodiscite-infectuse

251. Gouliouris T, Aliyu SH, Brown NM. Spondylodiscitis: update on diagnosis and management. Journal of Antimicrobial Chemotherapy [Internet]. 1 Nov 2010 [cited 3 Oct 2023];65(Supplement 3):iii11-24. Available from: https://academic.oup.com/jac/article-lookup/doi/10.1093/jac/dkq303

252. Stabler A, Reiser MF. Imaging of spinal infection. Radiol Clin North Am. Jan 2001;39(1):115-35.

253. Arkun R, Mete BD. Musculoskeletal brucellosis. SeminMusculoskeletRadiol. Nov 2011;15(5):470-9.

254. J.-J. Dubost JJD. EM-Consulte. [cited 5 Oct 2023]. Non-tuberculous infectious spondylodiscitis. Available at: https://www.em-consulte.com/article/50928/spondylodiscite-infectious-non-tuberculous.

255. Abid H, Chaabouni S, Frikha F, Toumi N, Souissi B, Lahiani D, et al. Contribution of imaging in the diagnosis of infectious sacroiliitis: about 19 cases. Pan Afr Med J [Internet]. 2014 Mar 6 [cited 2023 Oct 5];17:171. Available from: https://www.ncbi.nlm.nih.gov/pmc/articles/PMC4119445/

256. 1576619899.pdf [Internet]. [cited 5 Oct 2023]. Available from: https://www.infectiologie.org.tn/pdf_ppt_docs/recommandations/1576619899.p df

257. LECOUVET F, BOSMANS S, MALGHEM J, COSNARD G. Discovertebral, epidural and subdural infections. Feuillradiol. 2008;48(2):75-94.

258. Gorgülü A, Albayrak BS, Gorgülü E, Tural O, Karaaslan T, Oyar O, et al. Spinal epidural abscess due to Brucella. Surg Neurol. August 2006;66(2):141-6; discussion 146-147.

259. 10-ben_taarit-ben_maiz-.pdf [Internet]. [cited 5 Oct 2023]. Available from: http://actaorthopaedica.be/assets/33/10-ben_taarit-ben_maiz-.pdf

260. Lim KB, Kwak YG, Kim DY, Kim YS, Kim JA. Back Pain Secondary to Brucella Spondylitis in the Lumbar Region. Ann Rehabil Med [Internet]. Apr 2012 [cited 5 Oct 2023];36(2):282-6. Available from: https://www.ncbi.nlm.nih.gov/pmc/articles/PMC3358688/

261. N. Without * NS*. EM-Consulte. [cited 5 Oct 2023]. Infection du rachis - Spondylodiscites. Available from: https://www.em-consulte.com/article/733581/infection-du-rachis-n-spondylodiscites

262. J D Colmenero JDC. Sci-Hub | Pyogenic sacroiliitis a comparison between paediatric and adult patients | 10.1093/rheumatology/kem201 [Internet]. [cited 5 Oct 2023]. Available from: https://sci-hub.hkvisa.net/10.1093/rheumatology/kem201

263. Marion Hermet. Sci-Hub | Infectioussacroiliitis: aretrospective, multicentre study of 39 adults | 10.1186/1471-2334-12-305 [Internet]. [cited Oct 5, 2023]. Disponible sur: https://sci-hub.hkvisa.net/10.1186/1471-2334-12-305

264. Sci-Hub | Septicsacroiliitis | 10.1016/s0049-0172(96)80010-2 [Internet]. [cited 5 Oct 2023]. Available from: https://sci-hub.hkvisa.net/10.1016/s0049-0172(96)80010-2

265. Joshi KB, Brinker RA. Fine needle diagnosis in lumbar osteomyelitis. SkeletalRadiol. 1983;10(3):173-5.

266. F. Loubes-Lacroix FLL. EM-Consulte. [cited 5 Oct 2023]. Diagnostic imaging of infectious spondylodiscitis. Available from: https://www.em-consulte.com/article/25509/references/imagerie-diagnostique-de-la-spondylodiscite-infectuse

267. Marti'nez-Chamorro E, Munoz A, Esparza J, Munoz MJ, Giangaspro E. Focal cerebral involvement by neurobrucellosis: pathological and MRI findings. Eur J Radiol. Jul 2002;43(1):28-30.

268. Sci-Hub | Solitary extra-axial posterior fossa abscess due to neurobrucellosis | 10.1016/s0967-5868(03)00152-8 [Internet]. [cited 5 Oct 2023]. Disponible sur: https://sci-hub.hkvisa.net/10.1016/s0967-5868(03)00152-8

269. Sci-Hub | An unusual case of ruptured distal anterior cerebral artery aneurysm associated with brucellosis | 10.1016/j.jinf.2004.08.029 [Internet]. [cited 5 Oct 2023]. Available from: https://sci-

hub.hkvisa.net/10.1016/j.jinf.2004.08.029

270. Al-Deeb S, Madkour MM. Chapter 13 - Neurobrucellosis. In: Madkour MM, editor. Brucellosis [Internet]. Butterworth-Heinemann; 1989 [cited 27 Sep 2023]. p. 160-79. Available from: https://www.sciencedirect.com/science/article/pii/B9780723609414500201

271. Sci-Hub | Neurological syndromes of brucellosis. | 10.1136/jnnp.51.8.1017 [Internet]. [cited 5 Oct 2023]. Available from: https://sci-

272. hub.hkvisa.net/10.1136/jnnp.51.8.1017

273. A. Awada AA. EM-Consulte. [cited 5 Oct 2023]. Progressive paraparesis and deafness with leukoencephalopathy revealing chronic neurobrucellosis. Available from: https://www.em- consulte.com/article/281967/figures/paraparesis-and-progressive-deafness-with-leuko-encephalopathy.

274. Dahouk SA, Schneider T, Jansen A, Nockler K, Tomaso H, Hagen RM, et al. Brucella endocarditis in prosthetic valves. Can J Cardiol [Internet]. 2006 Sep [cited 2023 Oct 5];22(11):971-4. Available from: https://www.ncbi.nlm.nih.gov/pmc/articles/PMC2570246/

275. Lang R, Dagan R, Potasman I, Einhorn M, Raz R. Failure of Ceftriaxone in the Treatment of Acute Brucellosis. ClinicalInfectiousDiseases [Internet]. Feb 1, 1992 [cited Oct 8, 2023];14(2):506-9. Available from: https://academic.oup.com/cid/article-lookup/doi/10.1093/clinids/14.2.506

276. Najwa Khuri-Bulos NKB. Sci-Hub | Relapse of brucellosis following ofloxacin therapy | 10.1016/s0163-4453(05)80021-0 [Internet]. [cited 8 Oct 2023]. Disponible sur: https://sci-hub.hkvisa.net/10.1016/s0163-4453(05)80021-0

277. Acocella G, Bertrand A, Beytout J, Durrande JB, Rodriguez JAG, Kosmidis J, et al. Comparison of three different regimens in the treatment of acute brucellosis: a multicenter multinational study. J AntimicrobChemother [Internet]. 1989 [cited 8 Oct 2023];23(3):433-9. Available from: https://academic.oup.com/jac/article-lookup/doi/10.1093/jac/23.3.433

278. Ariza J, Gudiol F, Pallares R, Viladrich PF, Rufi G, Corredoira J, et al. Treatment of Human Brucellosis with Doxycycline plus Rifampin or Doxycycline plus Streptomycin: A Randomized, Double-Blind Study. Ann Intern Med [Internet]. 1 Jul 1992 [cited 8 Oct 2023];117(1):25-30. Disponible sur: https://www.acpjournals.org/doi/10.7326/0003-4819-117-1-25

279. Bruno Arcos-Lahuerta BAL. EM-Consulte. [cited 23 sept 2023]. Osteoarticular manifestations of brucellosis. Available from: https://www.em-consulte.com/article/8233/manifestations-osteoarticulaires-de-la-brucellose
brucellose.pdf [Internet]. [cited 7 Sep 2023]. Available from: http://medecinetropicale.free.fr/cours/brucellose.pdf

280. Maurin M, Raoult D. Optimum Treatment of Intracellular Infection. Drugs [Internet]. 1 Jul 1996 [cited 8 Oct 2023];52(1):45-59. Disponible sur: https://doi.org/10.2165/00003495-199652010-00004

281. Ranjbar M. Treatment of Brucellosis. In: Updates on Brucellosis [Internet]. IntechOpen; 2015 [cited 12 Oct 2023]. Available from: https://www.intechopen.com/chapters/48725

282. Fantinato C, Garin-Bastuji B, Jacquier H, Raskine L, Delcey V, Albert D, et al. Recurrent Brucella melitensis infections in a patient of Turkish origin. Option/Bio [Internet]. Sep 1, 2011 [cited Oct 8, 2023];22(459):17-9. Available from: https://www.sciencedirect.com/science/article/pii/S099259451170839X

283. Brucellosis JFEC on, Organization WH, Nations F and AO of the U. Joint FAO/WHO Expert Committee on Brucellosis [meeting held in Geneva from 3 to 9 December 1963]: fourth report [Internet]. World Health Organization; 1964 [cited 8 Oct 2023]. Available from: https://iris.who.int/handle/10665/40605

284. Yousefi-Nooraie R, Mortaz-Hejri S, Mehrani M, Sadeghipour P. Antibiotics for treating human brucellosis. Cochrane Database Syst Rev. 17 Oct 2012;2012(10):CD007179.

285. Brucellosis JFEC on, Organization WH. Joint FAO/WHO Expert Committee on Brucellosis [meeting held in Geneva from 12 to 19 November 1985]: sixth report [Internet]. World Health Organization; 1986 [cited 8 Oct 2023]. Available from: https://iris.who.int/handle/10665/40202

286. Smith CC. Treatment of Human Brucellosis. Scott Med J [Internet]. July 1976 [cited 8 Oct 2023];21 (3):132-3. Disponible sur: http://journals.sagepub.com/doi/10.1177/003693307602100313

287. Skalsky K, Yahav D, Bishara J, Pitlik S, Leibovici L, Paul M. Treatment of human brucellosis: systematic review and meta-analysis of randomised controlled trials. BMJ [Internet]. 29 March 2008 [cited 12 Oct2023];336(7646):701-4. Available from: https://www.bmj.com/lookup/doi/10.1136/bmj.39497.500903.25

288. GLOWACKA P, ZAKOWSKA D, NAYLOR K, NIEMCEWICZ M, BIELAWSKA-DROZD A. Brucella - Virulence Factors, Pathogenesis and Treatment. Pol J Microbiol [Internet]. June 2018 [cited 12 Oct 2023];67(2):151-61. Available from: https://www.ncbi.nlm.nih.gov/pmc/articles/PMC7256693/

289. Agalar C, Usubutun S, Turkyilmaz R. Ciprofloxacin and Rifampicin Versus Doxycycline and Rifampicin in the Treatment of Brucellosis. European Journal of Clinical Microbiology & Infectious Diseases [Internet]. 1999 Sep 2 [cited 2023 Oct 8];18(8):535-8. Disponible sur: http://link.springer.com/10.1007/s100960050344

290. Akova M, Uzun O, Akalin HE, Hayran M, Unal S, Gür D. Quinolones in treatment of human brucellosis: comparative trial of ofloxacin-rifampin versus doxycycline-rifampin. Antimicrob Agents Chemother [Internet]. 1993 Sep [cited 2023 Oct 8];37(9):1831-4. Available from: https://journals.asm.org/doi/10.1128/AAC.37.9.1831

291. Solera J, Rodrîguez-Zapata M, Geijo P, Largo J, Paulino J, Saez L, et al. Doxycycline-rifampin versus doxycycline-streptomycin in treatment of human brucellosis due to Brucella melitensis. The GECMEI Group. Grupo de Estudio de Castilla-la Mancha de EnfermedadesInfecciosas. Antimicrob Agents Chemother [Internet]. 1995 Sep [cited 2023 Jan 3];39(9):2061-7. Available from: https://journals.asm.org/doi/10.1128/AAC.39.9.2061

292. Hasanain A, Mahdy R, Mohamed A, Ali M. A randomized, comparative study of dual therapy (doxycycline-rifampin) versus triple therapy (doxycycline- rifampin-levofloxacin) for treating acute/subacute brucellosis. Braz J Infect Dis [Internet]. May 1, 2016 [cited Oct 8, 2023];20(3):250-4. Available from: http://www.bjid.org.br/en-a-randomized-comparative-study-dual-articulo-S1413867016300460

293. Ranjbar M, Keramat F, Mamani M, Kia AR, Khalilian F o-sadad, Hashemi SH, et al. Comparison between doxycycline-rifampin-amikacin and doxycycline- rifampin regimens in the treatment of brucellosis. International Journal of InfectiousDiseases [Internet]. March 1, 2007 [cited Oct 8, 2023];11(2):152-6. Available from: https://www.ijidonline.com/article/S1201-9712(06)00062- 2/fulltext

294. SoKs Garda del Pozo J, Solera J. Systematic review and meta-analysis of randomized clinical trials in the treatment of human brucellosis. PLoS One. 2012;7(2):e32090.

295. Alavi SM, Alavi L. Treatment of brucellosis: a systematic review of studies in recent twenty years. Caspian J Intern Med. 2013;4(2):636-41.

296. Karabay O, Sencan I, Kayas D, §ahin I. Ofloxacin plus Rifampicin versus Doxycycline plus Rifampicin in the treatment of brucellosis: a randomized clinical trial [ISRCTN11871179]. BMC InfectiousDiseases [Internet]. 23 June 2004 [cited 8 Oct 2023];4(1):18. Available from: https://doi.org/10.1186/1471-2334-4-18

297. Molins A, Montalban J, Codina A. Parkinsonism in neurobrucellosis. Journal of Neurology, Neurosurgery&Psychiatry [Internet]. 1 Dec 1987 [cited 8 Oct 2023];50(12):1707-8. Available from: https://jnnp.bmj.com/lookup/doi/10.1136/jnnp.50.12.1707-a

298. ROLAIN JM, MAURIN M. Le traitement des brucelloses. Antibiotiques (Paris). 2000;2(2):101-9.

299. Sci-Hub | Treatment of human brucellosis with doxycycline and gentamicin. | 10.1128/aac.41.1.80 [Internet]. [cited 8 Oct 2023]. Available from: https://sci-hub.hkvisa.net/10.1128/aac.41.1.80

300. Sci-Hub | Efficacy of Gentamicin plus Doxycycline versus Streptomycin plus Doxycycline in the Treatment of Brucellosis in Humans | 10.1086/501359 [Internet]. [cited 8 Oct 2023]. Available from: https://sci- hub.hkvisa.net/10.1086/501359

301. Spinal brucellosis | Bone & Joint [Internet]. [cited Oct 8, 2023]. Disponible sur: https://boneandjoint.org.uk/article/10.1302/0301-620X.67B3.3997939

302. Pappas G, Seitaridis S, Akritidis N, Tsianos E. Treatment of brucella spondylitis: lessons from an impossible meta-analysis and initial report of efficacy of a fluoroquinolone-containing regimen. International Journal of Antimicrobial Agents [Internet]. nov 2004 [cited 8 Oct 2023];24(5):502-7. Available from: https://linkinghub.elsevier.com/retrieve/pii/S092485790400216X

303. Greenberg RN, Kennedy DJ, Reilly PM, Luppen KL, Weinandt WJ, Bollinger MR, et al. Treatment of bone, joint, and soft-tissue infections with oral ciprofloxacin. Antimicrob Agents Chemother [Internet]. feb 1987 [cited Oct 8, 2023];31(2):151-5. Available from: https://journals.asm.org/doi/10.1128/AAC.31.2.151

304. Greenberg RN, Newman MT, Shariaty S, Pectol RW. Ciprofloxacin, Lomefloxacin, or Levofloxacin as Treatment for Chronic Osteomyelitis. Antimicrob Agents Chemother [Internet]. Jan 2000 [cited Oct 8, 2023];44(1):164-6. Available from: https://journals.asm.org/doi/10.1128/AAC.44.1.164-166.2000

305. Rissing JP. Antimicrobial Therapy for Chronic Osteomyelitis in Adults: Role of the Quinolones. CLIN INFECT DIS [Internet]. Dec 1997 [cited Oct 8, 2023];25(6):1327-33. Available from: https://academic.oup.com/cid/article-lookup/doi/10.1086/516150

306. Solera J, Martinez-Alfaro E, Espinosa A. Recognition and Optimum Treatment of Brucellosis: Drugs [Internet]. Feb 1997 [cited 23 Jan 2023];53(2):245-56. Disponible sur: http://link.springer.com/10.2165/00003495-199753020-00005

307. Solera J, Rodrîguez-Zapata M, Geijo P, Largo J, Paulino J, Saez L, et al. Doxycycline-rifampin versus doxycycline-streptomycin in treatment of human brucellosis due to Brucella melitensis. The GECMEI Group. Grupo de Estudio de Castilla-la Mancha de EnfermedadesInfecciosas. Antimicrob Agents Chemother. Sept 1995;39(9):2061-7.

308. Solera J, Paulino J, Rodrïguez-Zapata M, Medrano F, Geijo P, Jiménez F, et al [Brucellar sacroiliitis. A detailed review with an analysis of treatment efficacy. Rev Clin Esp. June 1, 1992;191(1):13-8.

309. Luna-Martinez JE, Mej^a-Teran C. Brucellosis in Mexico: current status and trends. Vet Microbiol. 2002 Dec 20;90(1-4):19-30.

310. O. Heinzlef E. EM-Consulte. [cited 8 oct 2023]. Acute myelopathies. Available at: https://www.em-consulte.com/article/36507/myelopathies- acute

311. Legrand E, Massin P, Levasseur R, Hoppé E, Chappard D, Audran M. Diagnostic strategy and therapeutic principles during infectious bacterial spondylodiscitis. Revue du Rhumatisme [Internet]. Apr 1, 2006 [cited Oct 8, 2023];73(4):373-9. Available from: https://www.sciencedirect.com/science/article/pii/S1169833006000767

312. Faria F, Viegas F. Spinal brucellosis: a personal experience of nine patients and a review of the literature. Spinal Cord [Internet]. May 1995 [cited 8 Oct 2023];33(5):294-5. Available from: https://www.nature.com/articles/sc199566

313. Ugarriza LF, Porras LF, Lorenzana LM, Rodrîguez-Sanchez JA, Garœ-Yagüe LM, Cabezudo JM. Brucellar spinal epidural abscesses. Analysis of eleven cases. British Journal of Neurosurgery [Internet]. Jan 2005 [cited Oct 8, 2023];19(3):235-40. Disponible sur: http://www.tandfonline.com/doi/full/10.1080/02688690500204949

314. Chelli Bouaziz M, Ladeb MF, Chakroun M, Chaabane S. Spinal brucellosis: a review. SkeletalRadiol [Internet]. Sept 2008 [cited Oct 8, 2023];37(9): 785-90. Disponible sur: http://link.springer.com/10.1007/s00256-007-0371-x

315. Ribeira T, Veiros I, Nunes R, Martins L. Experiência de Cinco Anos de um Serviço de Reabilitaçao. Acta Med Port.

316. 1.pdf [Internet]. [cited 8 Oct 2023]. Available from: https://www.sims-asso.org/uploads/pdfs/monographies/10/1.pdf

317. Ariza J, Gudiol F, Valverde J, Pallares R, Fernandez-Viladrich P, Rufi G, et al. Brucellar Spondylitis: A Detailed Analysis Based on Current Findings. Clinical Infectious Diseases [Internet]. 1985 Sep 1 [cited 2023 Oct 8];7(5):656-64. Available from: https://academic.oup.com/cid/article- lookup/doi/10.1093/clinids/7.5.656

318. al-Sibai MB, Halim MA, el-Shaker MM, Khan BA, Qadri SM. Efficacy of ciprofloxacin for treatment of Brucella melitensis infections. Antimicrob Agents Chemother [Internet]. 1992 Jan [cited 2023 Oct 8];36(1):150-2. Available from: https://www.ncbi.nlm.nih.gov/pmc/articles/PMC189243/

319. Pappas G, Christou L, Akritidis N, Tsianos EV. Quinolones for brucellosis: treating old diseases with new drugs. Clinical Microbiology and Infection [Internet]. 2006 Sep [cited 2023 Oct 8];12(9):823-5. Available from: https://linkinghub.elsevier.com/retrieve/pii/S1198743X14642993

320. Al-Orainey IO, Laajam MA, Al-Aska AK, Rajapakse CN. Brucella meningitis. J Infect. March 1987; 14(2):141-5.

321. Pascual J, Combarros O, Polo JM, Berciano J. Localized CNS brucellosis: report of 7 cases. Acta Neurologica Scandinavica. Oct 1988;78(4):282-9.

322. Karsen H, Tekin Koruk S, Duygu F, Yapici K, Kati M. Review of 17 cases of neurobrucellosis: clinical manifestations, diagnosis, and management. Arch Iran Med. August 2012;15(8):491-4.

323. Ceran N, Turkoglu R, Erdem I, Inan A, Engin D, Tireli H, et al. Neurobrucellosis: clinical, diagnostic, therapeutic features and outcome. Unusual clinical presentations in an endemic region. Braz J Infect Dis. 2011;15(1):52-9.

324. Sci-Hub | Multivariate model for predicting relapse in human brucellosis | 10.1016/s0163-4453(98)93342-4 [Internet]. [cited 8 Oct 2023]. Disponible sur: https://sci-hub.hkvisa.net/10.1016/s0163-4453(98)93342-4

325. Bodur H, Erbay A, Akinci E, Cj olpan A, Cj evik MA, Balaban N. Neurobrucellosis in an Endemic Area of Brucellosis. Scandinavian Journal of InfectiousDiseases [Internet]. feb 2003 [cited 8 Oct 2023];35(2):94-7. Disponible sur: http://www.tandfonline.com/doi/full/10.1080/0036554021000027000

326. Sci-Hub | Ear involvement in human brucellosis |

10.1017/s0022215100096705 [Internet]. [cited Oct 8, 2023]. Disponible sur: https://sci-hub.hkvisa.net/10.1017/s0022215100096705

327. McLean DR, Russell N, Khan MY. Neurobrucellosis: Clinical and Therapeutic Features. Clinical Infectious Diseases. 1 Oct 1992;15(4):582-90.

328. Mills SA. Surgical Management of Infective Endocarditis: Annals of Surgery [Internet]. Apr 1982 [cited Oct 8, 2023];195(4):367-83. Disponible sur: http://journals.lww.com/00000658-198204000-00001

329. Sci-Hub | Surgicaltreatment of brucella endocarditis | 10.1016/s0003-4975(00)02663-1 [Internet]. [cited 8 Oct 2023]. Available from: https://sci-hub.hkvisa.net/10.1016/s0003-4975(00)02663-1

330. Sunar H, Duran E. Vegetectomy in brucella endocarditis. The Annals of Thoracic Surgery [Internet]. 2002 Jun 1 [cited 2023 Oct 9];73(6):2036. Available from: https://www.annalsthoracicsurgery.org/article/S0003- 4975(02)03442-2/fulltext

331. Caldarera I, Albanese S, Piovaccari G, Ferlito M, Galli R, Squadrini F, et al [Brucella endocarditis: role of drug treatment associated with surgery]. Cardiologia. May 1996;41(5):465-7.

332. Hadjinikolaou L, Triposkiadis F, Zairis M, Chlapoutakis E, Spyrou P. Successful management of Brucellamellitensis endocarditis with combined medical and surgical approach. European Journal of Cardio-Thoracic Surgery [Internet]. June 2001 [cited 9 Oct 2023];19(6):806-10. Available from: https://academic.oup.com/ejcts/article-lookup/doi/10.1016/S1010-7940(01)00696-0

333. Lahdhili H, Ziadi M, Abdelmoulah S, Bey M, Ben Youssef A, Chenik S, et al [Brucella endocarditis of native valves. Report of 3 cases]. Tunis Med. Oct 2001;79(10):540-3.

334. Leandro J. Brucella endocarditis of the aortic valve. European Journal of Cardio-Thoracic Surgery [Internet]. 1998 Jan [cited 2023 Oct 9];13(1):95-7. Available from: https://academic.oup.com/ejcts/article- lookup/doi/10.1016/S1010-7940(97)00296-0

335. Uddin MJ, Sanyal SC, Mustafa AS, Mokaddas EM, Salama AL, Cherian G, et al. The role of aggressive medical therapy along with early surgical intervention in the cure of Brucella endocarditis. Ann Thorac Cardiovasc Surg. August 1998;4(4):209-13.

336. Ozkokeli M, Sensoz Y, Kayacioglu I, Akcar M, Erdem I, Gercekoglu H, et al. Treatment of Brucella Endocarditis: Our Surgical Experience with 6 Patients. The Heart Surgery Forum [Internet]. 7 Jul 2005 [cited 9 Oct 2023];8(4):E262-5. Available from: https://journal.hsforum.com/index.php/HSF/article/view/323

337. Ozsoyler i, Yilik L, Bozok §, El S, Emrecan B, Biçeroglu S, et al. Brucella Endocarditis: The Importance of Surgical Timing After Medical Treatment (Five Cases). Progress in Cardiovascular Diseases [Internet]. Jan 1, 2005 [cited Oct 9, 2023];47(4):226-9. Available from: https://www.sciencedirect.com/science/article/pii/S0033062004000799

338. Murdaca G, Colombo BM, Caiti M, Cagnati P, Massa G, Puppo F. Remission of brucella endocarditis in a patient with mitral valve mechanical prosthesis by antibiotic therapy alone: A case report. International Journal of Cardiology [Internet]. Apr 2007 [cited Oct 9, 2023];117(1):e35-6. Available from: https://linkinghub.elsevier.com/retrieve/pii/S0167527307000423

339. Jia B, Zhang F, Pang P, Zhang T, Zheng R, Zhang W, et al. Brucella endocarditis: Clinical features and treatment outcomes of 10 cases from Xinjiang, China. Journal of Infection [Internet]. may 2017 [cited Oct 9, 2023];74(5):512-4. Available from: https://linkinghub.elsevier.com/retrieve/pii/S0163445317300300

340. Raju, I. Tammi R I Ta. Sci-Hub | Brucella endocarditis - A series of five case reports | 10.1016/j.ihj.2012.12.017 [Internet]. [cited Oct 9, 2023]. Available from: https://sci-hub.hkvisa.net/10.1016/j.ihj.2012.12.017

341. Al-Harthi SS. The morbidity and mortality pattern of Brucella endocarditis. International Journal of Cardiology [Internet]. dec 1989 [cited Oct 9, 2023];25(3):321-4. Available from: https://linkinghub.elsevier.com/retrieve/pii/0167527389902222

342. Naoki Kawakami NK. Sci-Hub | Chronic Brucellosis in Japan | 10.2169/internalmedicine.2961-19 [Internet]. [cited Oct 9, 2023]. Available from: https://sci-hub.hkvisa.net/10.2169/internalmedicine.2961-19

343. Salehi M, Farbod F, Khalili H, Rahmani H, Jafari S, Abbasi A. Comparing efficacy and safety of high-dose and standard-dose rifampicin in the treatment of brucellosis: a randomized clinical trial. Journal of Antimicrobial Chemotherapy [Internet]. Apr 4, 2023 [cited Oct 9, 2023];78(4):1084-91. Available from: https://doi.org/10.1093/jac/dkad051

344. 4th International Meeting on the control of Neglected Zoonotic Diseases [Internet]. [cited 10 Oct 2023]. Available from: https://www.who.int/news/item/24-11-2014-4th-international-meeting-on-the- control-of-neglected-zoonotic-diseases

345. Brucellosis in humans and animals [Internet]. [cited 10 Oct 2023]. Available from: https://www.who.int/publications-detail-redirect/9789241547130

346. Pappas G, Papadimitriou P, Akritidis N, Christou L, Tsianos EV. The new global map of human brucellosis. The Lancet Infectious Diseases. 1 Feb 2006;6(2):91-9.

347. Franco MP, Mulder M, Gilman RH, Smits HL. Human brucellosis. The Lancet InfectiousDiseases [Internet]. 1 Dec 2007 [cited 11 Oct 2023];7(12):775-86.

348. Available at: https://www.thelancet.com/journals/laninf/article/PIIS1473-3099(07)70286-4/fulltext Gr HT. Preventive and Control Programs for Brucellosis in Human and Animals.

349. Adone R, Pasquali P. Epidemiosurveillance of brucellosis. Rev Sci Tech [Internet]. 1 Apr 2013 [cited 10 Oct 2023];32(1):199-205. Available from: https://doi.org/10.20506/rst.32.1.2202

350. Maurin M. Brucellosis at the dawn of the 21st century. Médecine et Maladies Infectieuses [Internet]. Jan 2005 [cited 3 Jan 2023];35(1):6-16. Available from: https://linkinghub.elsevier.com/retrieve/pii/S0399077X04002574

351. Aubrun F. RFE GERIATRICS / CERVICAL FRACTURE:4.

352. News from the Field. Am J Public Health Nations Health. Apr 1951;41(4):488-XLI.

353. Valette L. Medical prophylaxis of animal brucellosis. Revue d'élevage et de médecine vétérinaire des pays tropicaux [Internet]. 1 Apr 1987 [cited 10 Oct 2023];40(4):351-64. Available from: https://revues.cirad.fr/index.php/REMVT/article/view/8625

354. Marmonier A. Epidemiological and prophylactic study of animal and human brucellosis in a rural commune of Trièves: interest of the immunofluorescence reaction. 1974;

355. Garin-Bastuji M, Benzerrak M, Laval M. M. BODIN M. BERTAGNOLI.

356. Blasco JM, Diaz R. Brucella melitensis Rev-1 vaccine as a cause of human brucellosis. The Lancet [Internet]. 1993 Sep [cited 2023 Oct 10];342(8874):805. Available from: https://linkinghub.elsevier.com/retrieve/pii/014067369391571З

357. Brucella abortus Cyclic p-1,2-Glucan Mutants Have Reduced Virulence in Mice and Are Defective in Intracellular Replication in HeLa Cells | Infection and Immunity [Internet]. [cited 10 Oct 2023]. Available from: https://journals.asm.org/doi/full/10.1128/iai.69.7.4528-4535.2001

358. Sangari FJ, Grille MJ, De BagüésMariaPJ, Gonzalez-Carrero MI, Garœ-Lobo JM, Blasco JoséM, et al. The defect in the metabolism of erythritol of the Brucella abortus B19 vaccine strain is unrelated with its attenuated virulence in mice. Vaccine [Internet]. 1 Oct 1998 [cited 10 Oct 2023];16(17):1640-5. Available from: https://www.sciencedirect.com/science/article/pii/S0264410X98000632

359. Sangari FJ, Garœ-Lobo JM, Agüero J. The Brucella abortus vaccine strain B19 carries a deletion in the erythritol catabolic genes. FEMS MicrobiologyLetters [Internet]. Sep 1, 1994 [cited Oct 10, 2023];121(3):337-42. Disponible sur: https://doi.org/10.1111/j.1574-6968.1994.tb07123.x

360. Sangari F, Agüero J. Molecular basis of Brucella pathogenicity: an update. Microbiologi'a (Madrid, Spain). 1 Jul 1996;12:207-18.

361. Lounes N. History of bovine brucellosis screening and prophylaxis in Algeria. 2009.

362. Brucellosis JFEC on, Organization WH, Nations F and AO of the U. Joint FAO/WHO Expert Committee on Brucellosis [met at Geneva, June 29-July 6, 1970]: fifth report [Internet]. World Health Organization; 1971 [cited 11 Oct 2023]. Available from: https://iris.who.int/handle/10665/38126

363. Benkirane A. [Epidemiologic surveillance and prevention of brucellosis in ruminants: the example of the north African region and the Near East]. Revue scientifique et technique (International Office of Epizootics). 1 Jan 2002;20:757-67.

364. Chapter 8 SURVEILLANCE OF OVINE AND CAPRINE BRUCELLOSIS (excluding Brucella ovis infection) [Internet]. [cited 11 Oct 2023]. Available from: https://www.fao.org/3/Y4723E/y4723e0a.htm

365. Avila-Granados LM, Garcia-Gonzalez DG, Zambrano-Varon JL, Arenas-Gamboa AM. Brucellosis in Colombia: Current Status and Challenges in the Control of an Endemic Disease. Frontiers in Veterinary Science [Internet]. 2019 [cited 10 Oct 2023];6. Available from: https://www.frontiersin.org/articles/10.3389/fvets.2019.00321

366. Khurana SK, Sehrawat A, Tiwari R, Prasad M, Gulati B, Shabbir MZ, et al. Bovine brucellosis - a comprehensivereview. Vet Q [Internet]. [cited 10 Oct 2023];41(1):61-88. Available from: https://www.ncbi.nlm.nih.gov/pmc/articles/PMC7833053/

367. Zinsstag J, Roth F, Orkhon D, Chimed-Ochir G, Nansalmaa M, Kolar J, et al. A model of animal-human brucellosis transmission in Mongolia. Preventive Veterinary Medicine [Internet]. June 2005 [cited 10 Oct 2023];69(1-2):77-95. Available from: https://linkinghub.elsevier.com/retrieve/pii/S0167587705000577

368. In search of a combined brucellosis and tuberculosis vaccine for cattle [Internet]. [cited 10 Oct 2023]. Available from: https://www.scielo.cl/scielo.php?script=sci_arttext&pid=S0719-81322021000100001

369. Proces verba sa.pdf [Internet]. [cited 10 Oct 2023]. Available from: http://www.iresa.agrinet.tn/pdfs/Proces%20verba%20sa.pdf

370. Décret n° 2009-2200 fixant la nomenclature des maladies animales réglementées et édictant les mesures générales applicables à ces maladies. | FAOLEX [Internet]. [cited 10 Oct 2023]. Available from: https://www.fao.org/faolex/results/details/fr/c/LEX-FAOC093176/

371. B. Lopes L, Nicolino R, P. A. Haddad J. Brucellosis - Risk Factors and Prevalence: A Review. The Open Veterinary Science Journal [Internet]. 2010 [cited 10 Oct 2023];4(1). Available from: https://benthamopen.com/ABSTRACT/TOVSJ-4-72

372. index.pdf [Internet]. [cited 10 Oct 2023]. Available from: http://www.pasteur.tn/index.php?option=com_docman&task=doc_view&gid=880&tmpl=component&format=raw&Itemid=

373. hichem. IPT SEMINAR (February 9, 2023) Brucellosis: a re-emerging health risk [Internet]. [cited 10 oct 2023]. Available from: http://www.pasteur.tn/index.php?option=com_content&view=article&id=882:seminaire-de-lipt-9-fevrier-2023-la-brucellose--un-risque-sanitaire-re-emergent&catid=41:actualites&Itemid=147

Table of contents

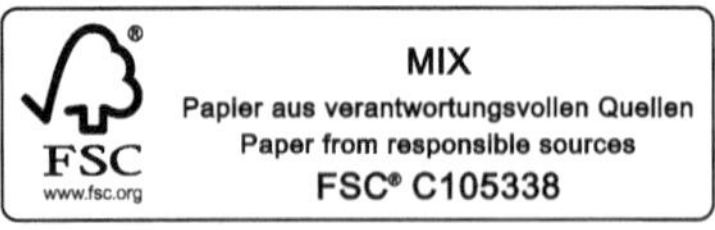

Printed by Books on Demand GmbH, Norderstedt / Germany